PASSION AND PATHOLOGY
IN VICTORIAN FICTION

Passion and Pathology
in Victorian Fiction

JANE WOOD

OXFORD
UNIVERSITY PRESS

OXFORD

UNIVERSITY PRESS

Great Clarendon Street, Oxford OX2 6DP

Oxford University Press is a department of the University of Oxford.
It furthers the University's objective of excellence in research, scholarship,
and education by publishing worldwide in

Oxford New York

Athens Auckland Bangkok Bogotá Buenos Aires
Cape Town Chennai Dar es Salaam Delhi Florence Hong Kong Istanbul
Karachi Kolkata Kuala Lumpur Madrid Melbourne Mexico City Mumbai
Nairobi Paris São Paulo Singapore Taipei Tokyo Toronto Warsaw
with associated companies in Berlin Ibadan

Oxford is a registered trade mark of Oxford University Press
in the UK and in certain other countries

Published in the United States
by Oxford University Press Inc., New York

© Jane Wood 2001

The moral rights of the author have been asserted
Database right Oxford University Press (maker)

First published 2001

British Library Cataloguing in Publication Data
Data available

Library of Congress Cataloging-in-Publication Data
Wood, Jane, 1943–
Passion and pathology in Victorian fiction/Jane Wood
p. cm.
Includes bibliographical references (p.) and index.
1. English fiction—19th century—History and criticism. 2. Body, Human, in literature.
3. Literature and medicine—Great Britain—History—19th century. 4. Neurology—Great
Britain—History—19th century. 5. Mental illness in literature. 6. Mind and body in
literature. 7. Emotions in literature. 8. Diseases in literature. I. Title.
PR878.B63 W66 2001   823´.809356—dc21   2001021215
ISBN 0-19-818760-2
ISBN 0-19-924713-7 (pbk.)

1 3 5 7 9 10 8 6 4 2

Typeset in Sabon by
Cambrian Typesetters, Frimley, Surrey

Printed in Great Britain
on acid-free paper by
Biddles Ltd,
Guildford and King's Lynn

In loving memory of my mother

Acknowledgements

In researching and writing this book I have received the invaluable assistance of many people. I wish to thank Sally Shuttleworth for sowing the seeds of my fascination with the subject in the first place and for her subsequent careful reading of an early version of the typescript. I am especially grateful to Inga-Stina Ewbank, who was unfailingly generous with her time and her knowledge during the course of my research. My thanks are due also to Coral Ann Howells and Gail Marshall for comments and queries which helped me to clarify arguments at a crucial stage of my project. I owe a particular debt to Helen Small, who read the typescript with meticulous attention and whose detailed comments, criticisms, and suggestions have greatly strengthened this book. To Francis O'Gorman, Paul Hammond, and David Lindley I express my gratitude for their very helpful comments on specific chapters, and to Cathy Tingle for directing me to a reference in G. H. Lewes's work which I would otherwise have overlooked. I thank all my colleagues and friends at the School of English, University of Leeds, for their encouragement and advice, and the staff of the following libraries for their assistance: the Brotherton Library, the Leeds Library, the University of Leeds Medical Library (now Health Sciences), the Wellcome Institute Library, London, Dr Williams's Library, London. Last, but not least, I wish to thank my family for their much-needed and often called-upon patience and support.

J.W.
Leeds
October 2000

Contents

Introduction

> It is to this physical constitution that we may attribute the
> gradual development of our various passions, many of our
> morbid appetites, and our unruly desires; according to our
> greater or less *susceptibility* or *impressionability* in our
> social relations, and the influence of our mental powers in
> checking and subduing their exigencies.[1]

As the title of this book suggests, Victorian fiction writers were
active participants in the discourses of medical science. That
they engaged in debates about health and disease is, at one level,
scarcely surprising. The constant reality of sickness and the
increasing incursion of medicine's authority into broader areas
of intellectual and social life were at once observable facts and
the tools of representation. *Passion and Pathology*, however, is
not about sickroom scenes, nor is it concerned to reveal doctors
as the tyrannical overlords of middle-class and mainly women's
lives: both are subjects with established places in nineteenth-
century literary and cultural criticism. It is scarcely necessary—
and indeed it is perhaps to risk cliché—to point out that
scientific explanations of human experience of the world rose to
a new prominence in the nineteenth century at the expense of
religious and philosophical ones. Nevertheless, as this book
aims to demonstrate, it is the case that the medical arguments
about the nature of the relationship between the physical,
mental, and social aspects of men's and women's lives raised
questions with which other thinkers and writers were continually preoccupied. Medicine and literature looked to each other
for elucidation and illustration. This is not to say that beliefs
and attitudes simply passed between them in a mutually
confirming continuity. One of the purposes of this book is to

---

[1] J. G. Millingen, *Mind and Matter, Illustrated by Considerations on Heredity,
Insanity, and the Influence of Temperament in the Development of the Passions*
(London: H. Hurst, 1847), p. 51.

examine the ambivalences and the points of contention which were not just by-products—the inevitable fallout—of the exchange of ideas, but were consciously addressed by medical writers and novelists alike. There are times when medical ideas and practices are simply used to reinforce existing prejudices and assumptions, and there are times, too, when wider questions about the moral and social implications of those ideas and practices are already begged by the limitations of the medical discourse itself. But the medical writers cited in this book, by far the majority eminent in their respective fields, all move beyond the particulars of their specialisms to ponder weighty ethical and philosophical questions raised by their scientific observations. William Carpenter, Thomas Laycock, and Henry Maudsley are three examples of doctors whose treatises on cerebral and neurological functioning slid almost imperceptibly— and, in Maudsley's case, in spite of his positivist principles—into elegant disquisitions on the nature of consciousness and the elusive relationship of body and mind.

In both literary and medical writings, representations of disorders such as neurosis, morbid consciousness, and neurasthenia encode meanings which reach beyond the sphere of medicine. Many of the novelists whose work I discuss here fostered a substantial intellectual interest in medical and related scientific matters. They read widely, not only to give scientific credibility to their work but to develop, and often challenge, fundamental premisses or the interpretations drawn from them. As Sally Shuttleworth has recently argued, Charlotte Brontë's fiction is not so much the work of 'an intuitive genius' as that of someone directly in touch with medical matters and with their political and economic ramifications.[2] Wilkie Collins certainly exploited the fictional possibilities of associational psychology and theories of the interpretation of dreams but, at the same time, his writing is well informed on current research into complex issues such as the brain's unconscious activity and the mysterious processes of the mind.[3] George Eliot's familiarity with scientific

[2] Sally Shuttleworth, *Charlotte Brontë and Victorian Psychology* (Cambridge: Cambridge University Press, 1996), p. 1.

[3] See Jenny Bourne Taylor, *In the Secret Theatre of Home: Wilkie Collins, Sensation Narrative, and Nineteenth-Century Psychology* (London: Routledge, 1988).

theories is well known. Her use of medical paradigms to explore the truth values of different forms of knowledge as well as the interrelations of individuals and social structures has been intricately examined.[4] Towards the end of the century, Thomas Hardy's writing is charged with tensions specific to the age but, as critics have shown, those very tensions are thrown into sharp relief by his own research into specialized topics such as the mechanisms of heredity and nervous degeneration.[5] By giving similar consideration to contextualizing literary texts with the scientific theories which have informed them, this book maintains that, far from writing in an isolated realm of the imagination, novelists are critically engaged in medicine's search for understanding of the complex processes governing emotional and sensory experience.

Neurology is the branch of medicine that is central to the arguments of this book.[6] The idea of a physical mechanism for explaining psychological states was a compelling one which suited a positivist age. To the lay mind, it seemed logical that the nervous system formed the vital bridge between the body's sensations and the mind's consciousness of them. Neurophysiologists, moreover, were confident that it was the mediating properties of the nervous system which explained how invisible impulses translated into human action and behaviour. On a less exalted plane, nervous disorder was a dominant category of Victorian disease narratives. As early as 1807, Thomas Trotter unhesitatingly affirmed that '*nervous disorders* have now taken the place of fevers, and may be justly reckoned two thirds of the whole, with which civilized society is afflicted'.[7] Matthew Arnold speaks of nervous exhaustion as

[4] See, for example, Lawrence Rothfield, *Vital Signs: Medical Realism in Nineteenth-Century Fiction* (Princeton: Princeton University Press, 1992); Sally Shuttleworth, *George Eliot and Nineteenth-Century Science: The Make-Believe of a Beginning* (Cambridge: Cambridge University Press, 1984).

[5] See especially William Greenslade, *Degeneration, Culture and the Novel 1880–1940* (Cambridge: Cambridge University Press, 1994).

[6] The impact of the science of neurology on all branches of nineteenth-century medicine and on wider sociological, ethical, and general cultural issues has been exhaustively researched by Janet Oppenheim. See '*Shattered Nerves': Doctors, Patients, and Depression in Victorian England* (New York: Oxford University Press, 1991).

[7] Thomas Trotter, *A View of the Nervous Temperament, Being a Practical Enquiry into the Increasing Prevalence, Prevention, and Treatment of Those*

'this strange disease of modern life', and even the centuries-old trope of love-sickness is accommodated to the new neuroscience when Arthur Symons observes that 'the modern malady of love is nerves'.[8] Few, according to Peter Gay, could fail to be sensible of a cultural phenomenon to which novelists, poets, doctors, artists, and philosophers so richly subscribed.[9] But if the phrase 'the century of nerves' has become a commonplace, it was one based on a reality of scientific and cultural change. By the closing years, the very word 'civilized' had been adapted to the claims of evolutionary discourse in its ground-breaking assertions of a biological model of development according to which the human nervous system had progressed from the primitive and instinctual to the hypersensitive and over-refined.

Within the broad category of neuropathology explored in this book are the range of illnesses known in the period as 'functional nervous disorders'.[10] Neither obviously organic nor exclusively mental, these afflictions were, by definition, disorders of function occurring in the connections between mental and bodily experience. Importantly, however, novelists were more concerned with the wider social meanings and the

Diseases Commonly Called Nervous (London: Longman, Hurst, Rees, Orme, and Brown, 1807), p. xvii, emphasis in original. For most medical observers (including Trotter) until the nineteenth century, 'civilized' predominantly meant 'leisured' society. Urban growth and industrialization added another dimension to nervous stress, but the existence of nervous disease among the working classes was largely ignored or denied.

[8] Matthew Arnold, 'The Scholar-Gipsy' (1853), in Kenneth Allott (ed.), *The Poems of Matthew Arnold* (London: Longmans, 1965). See also Arthur Symons, 'Nerves', in *London Nights* (1895), repr. in *The Faber Book of Twentieth Century Verse*, new edn., rev. by John Heath-Stubbs and David Wright (London: Faber, 1953).

[9] Peter Gay, *The Bourgeois Experience: Victoria to Freud*, 2 vols. (New York: Oxford University Press, 1986), ii. pp. 329–52.

[10] 'Functional nervous disorder' is the term more generally used in the nineteenth century for 'neurosis'. It refers to those diseases which were of nervous origin, but which revealed no structural changes to the brain or nervous system after death. Also, as W. F. Bynum points out, there is an important difference between so-called 'nervous diseases' and 'diseases of the nervous system'. In a reference to Moritz Romberg's *A Manual of the Nervous Diseases of Man*, 2nd edn., trans. by E. H. Sieveking, 2 vols. (London: Sydenham Society, 1853), Bynum describes Romberg's title as significant in that it defines 'a functional rather than structural outlook'. See 'The Nervous Patient in Eighteenth and Nineteenth-Century Britain: The Psychiatric Origins of British Neurology', in W. F. Bynum, Roy Porter, and Michael Shepherd (eds.), *The Anatomy of Madness: Essays in the History of Psychiatry*, 3 vols. (London: Tavistock Publications, 1985), i. pp. 89–102 (p. 92).

disputed interpretations of morbid states than they were with clinical accuracy. They were concerned, also, with questions of identity and with the implications for coherent selfhood of alienating nervous conditions. The first two chapters of *Passion and Pathology* consider the nervous symptoms of women and men, respectively, as signs and functions of the social, moral, sexual, or economic displacement of those who suffer them. When novelists constructed their heroes and heroines as anomalies in the dominant cultural order, they both highlighted and challenged the gendered assumptions upon which the norms of health and disease were established. Portrayals of individual women in fiction are examined in the light of the definitive pathologies of 'Woman' which, far from being confined to medical textbooks, were widely circulated through the general periodical. If women were designated as medical problems by their very nature, men were more likely to be pathologized by association. Thus, the nervously sensitive male was effectively feminized by a disorder which marginalized him socially, sexually, and psychologically from the prevailing norms of manliness. From representations of the effects of passionate excess—of emotion in women and of imagination in men—Chapter 3 turns to the relationship between physiology and consciousness. Beginning with the shared fascination of doctors and fiction writers for states of altered consciousness such as those experienced in delirium, the discussion is extended into the influential physiological arguments for the material basis of mental life. Finally, tensions arising from the findings of biologists and physicists on the subject of degeneration on familial and global scales, together with the economic and educational pressures of the last decade of the century, called for new formulations of disease. The specific concerns of the 1890s bore down upon definitions of female nervous illness and shifted the terms of age-old arguments about women's alleged natural inferiority onto the scientifically 'proven', but yet contradictory, categories of arrested development and over-refinement.

Historians of medicine and cultural historians have been invaluable to literary critics working in interdisciplinary fields: the former by setting events and developments in medicine in the wider contexts of social, moral, political, and economic changes; and the latter by showing how the cultural determinants of representation mean that it is no longer possible to think in terms of isolated, stable, and self-coherent forms of knowledge or to assume that one discursive system simply reflects another.[11] Since Michel Foucault advocated the critical interrogation of the 'objects' of history generally assumed to be natural formations, it has become almost intuitive to examine objects such as madness, medicine, punishment, sexuality, or the middle class, to give some examples, as having been constructed through particular genealogies and systems of knowledge. However, whilst it is true that the defining criteria of diseases were continually being revised in line with changing sensibilities, and whilst it is also true that doctors were at pains to validate their new-found professional authority, it is not my purpose in this book to claim, in a Foucauldian manner, that the changes served only to perpetuate the centrality of medicine as a dominant discourse.[12] Similarly, while feminist studies of Victorian medicine and its dealings with women have been helpful in drawing attention both to the high-handed interventionism of doctors into women's lives and to the policy of giving scientific sanction to absurdly prescriptive ideologies of femininity, many have presented a picture of an oppressive regime in which woman was always an anomaly, caught in the double-bind of victim or rebel. But on closer and more extensive reading of the published medical material it becomes clear that doctors were concerned first and

[11] Of the many medical histories, see Ilza Veith, *Hysteria: The History of a Disease* (Chicago: Chicago University Press, 1965); Roy Porter, *Mind-Forg'd Manacles: A History of Madness in England from the Restoration to the Regency* (Cambridge, Mass.: Harvard University Press, 1987); Edward Shorter, *From Paralysis to Fatigue: A History of Psychosomatic Illness in the Modern Era* (New York: Free Press, 1992); Janet Oppenheim, cited in n. 6 above; Charles E. Rosenberg, 'Body and Mind in Nineteenth-Century Medicine: Some Clinical Origins of the Neurosis Construct', *Bulletin of the History of Medicine*, 63 (1989), 185–97; and the collection of essays in *The Anatomy of Madness* as cited above. See Ludmilla Jordanova, *Sexual Visions: Images of Gender in Science and Medicine Between the Eighteenth and Twentieth Centuries* (Hemel Hempstead: Harvester Wheatsheaf, 1989); and Mary Jacobus, Evelyn Fox Keller and Sally Shuttleworth (eds.), *Body/Politics: Women and the Discourses of Science* (London: Routledge, 1990) for helpful readings in science and wider cultural discourse.
[12] For a different view of the medical profession's patriarchal authority, see Frank Mort, *Dangerous Sexualities: Medico-Moral Politics in England Since 1830* (London: Routledge, 1987).

foremost with understanding disease and healing their patients.[13]

Two recent studies which explore the links between medicine and fiction in nineteenth-century intellectual and imaginative life but which, one might argue, are positioned on opposite ends of the body/mind divide, so to speak, are Athena Vrettos's *Somatic Fictions* and Helen Small's *Love's Madness*. *Somatic Fictions* explores the extraordinarily ubiquitous preoccupation with the body in nineteenth-century medical and literary narrative. Vrettos argues that, for the Victorians, illness was much more than the reality that we read of in personal accounts of suffering; it was an imaginative construct for transforming 'the abstract into the concrete', for locating 'in the body the source of sexual and social divisions', thereby providing doctors and novelists with the narrative means for articulating wider social and cultural perplexities.[14] *Love's Madness* focuses on the sick mind rather than the body. By re-examining the representations, in fiction and in medicine, of the woman driven to insanity through the loss of her lovers, Small accounts for the transferability and repetition of images of the madwoman across disciplines at a time when sensibility and sentimentalism were giving way to a scientific realism.[15] Given that the epigraph opening this study places my book, medically speaking, between the two, conceptually, *Passion and Pathology* steps into a lively field of critical debate on nineteenth-century literature and medical science.

---

[13] The rather limited critiques appeared mainly during the 1970s. See, for example, Barbara Ehrenreich and Deirdre English, *Complaints and Disorders: The Sexual Politics of Sickness* (London: Writers and Readers Publishing Co-operative, 1976); and Sara Delamont and Lorna Duffin (eds.), *The Nineteenth-Century Woman: Her Cultural and Physical World* (London: Croom Helm, 1978). Though much more comprehensive, and historically focused, Elaine Showalter's *The Female Malady: Women, Madness, and English Culture, 1830–1980* (London: Virago, 1987. First published 1985) still tends to communicate a sense of outrage over attitudes and treatment which offend our later sensibilities.

[14] Athena Vrettos, *Somatic Fictions: Imagining Illness in Victorian Culture* (Stanford: Stanford University Press, 1995), p. 3.

[15] Helen Small, *Love's Madness: Medicine, the Novel, and Female Insanity, 1800–1865* (Oxford: Clarendon Press, 1996).

CHAPTER ONE

Nature's Invalids: The Medicalization of Womanhood

THE 'PROBLEM' OF WOMAN: INTERPRETATION AND THERAPEUTICS

This chapter is about mental causes and physical symptoms. Put less bluntly, it examines the ways in which a long recognized interrelation of body and mind was put to work to explain the baffling functional disorders of women. Predominantly, it is concerned with the correspondences and contradictions between the portrayals of individual women in fiction and the definitive pathologies of 'Woman'. Female invalids feature largely in Victorian texts and the aim of this chapter is to explore the extent to which, at a time when medical literature, however well meaning, habitually referred women's illnesses to the peculiarities of the female nature, fiction writers were affirming or contesting the essentializing assumptions of medical classification and interpretation.

New conceptualizations of psychosomatic disorders in women were hampered by decades, if not centuries, of explanations of hysteria. Old ideas were accommodated to new conditions, and representations of female sickness took the form they did because of the prevailing social, sexual-political, and economic conditions of the time. Many words have been written on the effects of a growing industrial economy on ideas of women's role and, by extension, of the social meanings of their illnesses. It may be that the complex equation of male and female, public and private, work and home, has been too readily simplified into the familiar model of separate gender spheres—the female private sphere of domesticity and the male public sphere of work. Nevertheless, the linking of women's well-being to contented domesticity was a concept which held considerable sway at the time, not only in middle-class advice literature but also in influential medical literature and social commentary. A historical development which had a significant impact on the cultural perception of womanhood was the professionalization of medicine. When doctors, from physicians to alienists to surgeons, organized themselves into professional bodies, they secured their authority as possessors of privileged knowledge.[1] Since the overwhelming majority of these professionals were men, male authority over female disorder was thus institutionalized. The sum of elements from popular myth and medical science was a perception of woman which seemed unproblematically to mingle a self-evidently idealized image of an 'angel in the house' and a reality of permanent invalidism.

The novelists Charlotte Brontë and Charles Dickens both work with culturally inscribed beliefs about femininity, female sexuality, and women's role in society. *Shirley* (1849) and *Little Dorrit* (1855–7) were published at a time when ideas about moral management and the centrality of doctrines of domestication were exerting a powerful force, not only in public institutions such as asylums but also in the social institutions of marriage and the home.[2] The idealization of woman as the morally pure, passive, 'angel in the house' worked to make a virtue of a social prescription and thereby served an expedient need. In the interests of preserving the almost exclusively masculine domains of science, industry, scholarship, and politics, the image of the willingly self-sacrificial 'angel' was appropriated and circulated with enthusiasm by moral philosophers, social theorists, artists, and scientists alike, contributing to the formulation of what was perhaps the most powerful and pervasive stereotype supporting the strategic notion of separate spheres.[3] This is not to suggest, however, that passive, angelic

[1] See M. Jeanne Peterson, *The Medical Profession in Mid-Victorian London* (Berkeley: University of California Press, 1978) for a detailed history.

[2] See Elaine Showalter, *The Female Malady: Women, Madness, and English Culture, 1830–1980* (London: Virago, 1987).

[3] The title of Coventry Patmore's poem, 'The Angel in the House' (1854–6), crystallized the idealizations into the familiar stereotype. John Ruskin's 'Of Queens' Gardens', frequently cited in support of the ideal, presents a somewhat misleading picture of Victorian middle-class collective identity when passages are extracted out of context. Ruskin's objective was, rather, to exhort women to use their alleged

self-sacrifice was taken to be necessarily the reality of the middle-class woman's life nor even the model to which she aspired. The complacent categorization of Victorian womanhood to virtuous domesticity fails to acknowledge the richness and diversity of either fictional representation or social practice. Indeed, the orthodox picture of domestic ideology, which served as a standard whereby women's conformity and resistance, health and disease could be measured, is vigorously asserted, negotiated, and contested in the range of writing across the period.

Charlotte Brontë's depiction of Caroline Helstone's ailing health brings to the fore a painful discrepancy between public expectation and private need. The constructed ideal of the endlessly enduring woman, excluded from the masculine world of industry and politics, but at the same time expected to be contentedly occupied with her supporting and caring role, is systematically dismantled as Brontë opposes the vision of romantic complementarity to the disappointing reality of Caroline's life. For Dickens, the representation of gender-specific roles, and the moral meanings which are attached to those roles, are inseparable. In Mrs Clennam and Miss Havisham we are presented with women whose passionate excess seems on the surface of things to parody the model of woman's confinement within the domestic sphere. But then the savagely punitive treatment which each receives at their creator's hand, far from ridiculing the prescriptive doctrines of womanhood, ultimately works to re-inscribe them. Although Dickens moves provocatively towards appearing to challenge the precepts underlying cultural representations of morbid femininity, he retreats into the conservative medical paradigms which equated social transgression with sickness.

In the period leading up to mid-century, doctors, philosophers, and social commentators were scarcely distinguishable from each other in the language they used to expatiate on

special attributes more publicly to improve what he saw to be a spiritually debased society: *Sesame and Lilies* (1865), 14th edn. (London: George Allen, 1894). An excellent revision of the ideology of separate spheres is Amanda Vickery's compellingly sceptical paper 'Golden Age to Separate Spheres? A Review of the Categories and Chronology of English Women's History', *The Historical Journal*, 36/2 (1993), 383–414.

women's innate suitability for their special social and moral function. Availing themselves of ready-made assumptions about women's nature, the spokesmen for separate spheres fused the temperamental and the physiological connotations of the concept of 'nature' and fixed women's social, moral, and emotional lives in biology. As the case for the determining power of biology gained strength from evolutionary science, nineteenth-century medicine took a lead in shaping a bourgeois economy which harnessed women to their bodies and necessitated their exclusion from the public domain. Whilst, as Amanda Vickery has rightly warned, the rhetoric should not be taken as evidence of the historical reality, it is nevertheless true that for numbers of middle-class women the gap between what was expected of them and their experience seemed to grow wider.

On the one hand, women were persuaded that nature clearly intended them for a spiritual role in social organization. John Elliotson is only one in a long line of physicians to draw upon literary precedent to formulate a feminine affective history:

[I]t is clear that woman is not intended for the rough business of the *world*, and that her perfection is best displayed in quiet intellectual and elegant occupations, and in care and activity directed to the happiness of those individuals to whom she is attached.

> 'For nothing lovelier can be found
> In woman, than to study household good,
> And good works in her husband to promote.'
> *Paradise Lost* (Book ix, 232).[4]

In confusing contrast to this rather ethereal image, women were assailed at every turn with the fact of their problematic physiology. The contradictions which they were obliged to negotiate are depressingly spelled out in treatise after treatise warning of the potential hazards in store for them throughout adult life. This late-century extract speaks ominously of the choice the female nervous patient must face, but its message is one which implicitly addresses all women:

---

[4] John Elliotson, *Human Physiology*, 5th edn. (London: Longmans, 1840), p. 700, emphasis in original.

If such a woman marries, she runs innumerable risks in pregnancy, childbirth, and lactation, and she is likely to have weakly children; if she remains single, she has nearly as many hazards in unused functions, hysteria, unsatisfied cravings, objectless emotion, and want of natural interests in life.[5]

A healthy woman could not reassure herself with reasoning that these warnings did not apply to her. The risks involved in pregnancy and childbirth spoke for themselves. But no woman could be assured of escaping since, if all the socio-medical theories were to be believed, she was already, by nature, predisposed to psychosomatic illness by virtue of the alleged morbid connection between her mental organization and physiology.

Hysteria, the archetypal female nervous disorder, rose to a new prominence in the nineteenth century as a condition whose clinical criteria could be modified in order to diagnose all the behaviours which did not fit the prescribed model of Victorian womanhood. Representations of disease and disorder proliferate and change according to contemporary attitudes, preconceptions, fashions, and assumptions, as much as to the specifics of medical knowledge. Ilza Veith has shown how, throughout history, this has been particularly true of hysteria, a disease whose symptoms are modified, not only by 'the state of medicine in general and the knowledge of the public about medical matters' but also by 'social expectancy, tastes, mores, and religion'.[6] Representations of hysterical disorder moved freely between the normal and the pathological, appropriating ideas and images from a whole range of often contradictory knowledges. Historical pronouncements on the role of the uterus, the brain, culture and heredity, the temperament, vapours, and literary and visual portrayals of pining, wilting women or madwomen, all contributed, with varying degrees of emphasis, to these representations.

Medical knowledge itself was eclectic, fluctuating between new and long-established theories, and constantly modifying its formulations to changing social and economic conditions.

[5] T. S. Clouston, *Clinical Lectures on Mental Diseases*, 2nd edn. (London: John Churchill, 1887), p. 44.

[6] Ilza Veith, *Hysteria: The History of a Disease* (Chicago: University of Chicago Press, 1965), p. 209.

In such a climate, the term 'hysteria' served both to encompass and mask the bewildering diversity of definitions and explanations, a catch-all word that blurred the distinctions between myth and methodology, fact and fiction, in a category acknowledged at the time as the most 'protean' of maladies.[7] Prevailing notions of sexual ideology coloured the way in which hysterical disorder was perceived, and inevitably mediated, in both medical and literary genres. Ideas of orthodox sexual behaviour, as well as ideals of masculinity and femininity, were important measures of what constituted the subversive, the deviant, the iconoclastic. With its vague and flexible symptoms, hysteria encompassed both excess and restraint, and defined at once the paroxysmal lapses of self-control and the frozen internality of suppression.

It is the capacity for containing such contradictions which gave to hysteria both a practical utility and a metaphorical instrumentality for representing the little understood processes of psychosomatic disorder. Above all, it provided an inclusive category for the phenomenon of psychological states manifesting as bodily symptoms. What is meant here is not exactly equivalent to the modern understanding of the dynamics of psychosomatic disease. Nor is it simply to reiterate the critical trope of the legible body which has so enabled modern insight into the theory and practice of Victorian psychology. As an interpretative tool the concept of the body as text, available for reading as a set of signs or a site of meaning, has become in many ways indispensable. My concern, however, is with emphasizing the ways in which the hysterical body was causally linked to the transgression of social and sexual prescriptions. In the context of psychosomatic medicine, the belief that psychological states, as well as wider cultural, social, sexual-political, and economic anxieties, left their indelible

---

7 John Conolly writes of hysteria how '[i]n different individuals, and in the same individual in different attacks, the disorder to which the name hysteria seems justly given . . . assumes shapes so various that it would be in vain to attempt to describe them all'. See J. Forbes, A. Tweedie, and J. Conolly, (eds.), *The Cyclopaedia of Practical Medicine*, 4 vols. (London: Sherwood, Gilbert, Piper *et al*, 1833–5), ii. pp. 557–86 (p. 560). See also Henry Maudsley, *Body and Mind: An Enquiry Into Their Connection and Mutual Influence, Specially in Reference to Mental Disorders*, being the Gulstonian Lectures for 1870 (London: Macmillan, 1870), p. 68.

marks on the body represents a crucial stage in a developing science. As will be seen in a later chapter, this process of inscription opens out to incorporate a more securely formulated understanding of the nervous system as the mediating mechanism between mind and body. But already, the notion of the body as a harbour of inexpressible emotional secrets accessible only by means of the specialized knowledge and interpretative skills of the practitioner is one which is both propounded and challenged in literary depictions of invalid women.

Brontë and Dickens each address gender hierarchy and social expectation, matters which are themselves products of the intersection of specifically medical and broadly ideological theorizing, in terms of signs upon the body. In both *Shirley* and *Little Dorrit*, the nuances of the psychological states of the two women at the centre of my discussion are articulated as bodily changes. Athena Vrettos has recently highlighted the ways in which 'women's emotional lives were perceived as both somatically encoded and medically or intuitively legible, as mysterious texts that defied interpretation at the same time they demanded it'. Vrettos rightly makes explicit the tension in Victorian texts (medical as well as fictional) that surrounded the problem of interpretation.[8] The idea of the female body as text, at once demanding to read and resisting reading, underlines important aspects of the gender dynamics with which fiction writers were concerned. Specifically, it draws attention to the physical consequences of social prescriptions of femininity as repressive quiescence and patient endurance. In the little known *Adela Cathcart* (1864), George MacDonald bases an entire novel on the process of reading and understanding the signs and symptoms on the body of the female sufferer. In the case of the eponymous heroine, as we shall see, the male observers and physician are less interested in the cause of Adela's life-threatening decline than they are in proving the efficacy of the singularly unusual method of cure. Charlotte Brontë, however, continually overturns gendered and hierarchized models of reading and interpretation. The matter of correct or incorrect reading of the signs of illness is

---

[8] Athena Vrettos, *Somatic Fictions: Imagining Illness in Victorian Culture* (Stanford: Stanford University Press, 1995), p. 29.

crucial, but not, as one might expect, as the preliminary to diagnosis and cure. Indeed, Brontë's narrative remains profoundly sceptical of the concept of the female body as a problem to be solved by some external agency, be that agency male or female.

When Caroline's uncle, Mr Helstone, is perplexed by the unaccountable changes in women's appearance: 'To-day you see them bouncing, buxom, red as cherries, and round as apples; to-morrow they exhibit themselves effete as dead weeds, blanched and broken down', he expresses a widely held male view of the woman's body as problematic; 'the puzzle' that must be solved.[9] Only two years after the publication of *Shirley*, an anonymous reviewer of Thomas Laycock's book, *A Treatise on the Nervous Diseases of Women*, echoes Helstone when he reiterates the difficulty faced by the male observer. It is, he writes, in respect of the mysterious correspondence between woman's 'psychological imperfections' and 'corporeal disorder and defect—that woman presents the most interesting problems for inquiry and solution'.[10] In this medical text, the role of the doctor is emphatically understood to be interpretative rather than therapeutic. '[I]t is only by a wide and comprehensively philosophical inquiry in the two directions indicated [body and mind]', the writer adds, 'that anything like a satisfactory comprehension of the problems can be acquired, or the problems themselves adequately solved'.[11] The prolix and so-called 'philosophical' excursus which follows is rooted in the belief in woman's problematic nature, but it is the task of the informed observer to interpret the nature of the problem, not necessarily to solve it. Brontë's challenges to these gendered medical paradigms leave many paradoxes in place. Not least of these was one which, for Brontë, as indeed for some physicians, pinpointed the dilemma at the centre of women's lives; namely the obligation to suppress or conceal emotion whilst recognizing restraint itself as the cause of ill health.

[9] Charlotte Brontë, *Shirley* (1849), ed. by Herbert Rosengarten and Margaret Smith (Oxford: Oxford University Press, 1979; with intro. by Margaret Smith, 1981), p. 189. Subsequent references to this edition will be given in the text.
[10] Anon., 'Woman in Her Psychological Relations', *Journal of Psychological Medicine and Mental Pathology*, 4 (1851), 18–50 (p. 21).
[11] 'Woman in Her Psychological Relations', p. 21.

The unlikely pairing of Brontë's Caroline Helstone and Dickens's Mrs Clennam is a reflection of the ways in which invalid narratives work with and against the ideological framework in which they are constructed. Each is informed by mid-Victorian medical representations of female psychosomatic illness as a function of social, moral, or sexual-political transgression. Perhaps not surprisingly, they engage rather differently with the tensions between scientifically authorized norms of femininity and women's knowledge of themselves. Brontë's portrayal of Caroline's illnesses articulates an anguished search for the truth of the causes and nature of female pathology. It negotiates with ideas of sickness as constitutional, and as a consequence of the seemingly doomed struggle with the contradiction between desire and the social (underwritten by medical) requirement to conceal it. Dickens takes an altogether more censorious view of the female invalid, and suggestively portrays states of health or infirmity in terms of an individual's willingness to subscribe to the cultural prescriptions of womanhood, and of the extent of her resistance to them. Where Brontë's scenes of sickness bring into focus the realities of women's experience measured against the myths, those of Dickens exaggerate the myths into parodic replications of separate-sphere ideology. The myths surrounding female nature were explanations proffered in response to the 'problem' which medical science had itself largely invented. For George MacDonald, the young female invalid with her unknown disease is constructed in terms of a social problem for the family, a problem resolved only by her reintegration into normal social functioning. The course of treatment prescribed, moreover, is designed to appeal to the sympathies and feelings believed to be inherent in a woman's nature.

Confident in their specialized knowledge, doctors set about the business of medicalizing gender and social spheres. The official view at the time is well represented in another passage from John Elliotson's *Human Physiology*, the medical textbook to which I have already referred and which was in its fifth edition in the 1840s. It is noteworthy for the particular reasons that it was a book which was in the Brontë household and that Elliotson himself was known to Dickens through their mutual interest in mesmerism, an enthusiasm which eventually cost the

eminent and highly respected clinician his professional post.[12]
For a medical textbook, *Human Physiology* is rich in literary
allusion, philosophical speculation, and cultural preconception.
It is revealing how the subject of female physiology prompts the
expression of a torrent of opinion, assumption, and value judgement that is conspicuously absent from the rest of the book. The
following passage is by no means untypical of the way in which
doctors ascribed meanings to physiological difference which
went far beyond clinical necessity and the limits of their diagnostic responsibility. Having waxed lyrical about the suitability
of woman's 'corporeal structure' for the procreative and
parental duties she must undertake, Elliotson explains:

Greatly inferior to man in reasoning powers, extent of views, originality and grandeur of conception, as well as in corporeal strength,
woman possesses more acuteness of external sensation, of apprehension, and of emotion, though a smaller range of intelligence and less
permanence of impression, more tenderness, affection, and compassion, more of all that is endearing and capable of soothing human
woes; but less consistency, impetuosity, courage, and firmness of character, except where affection subsists. She is more disposed to believe
all things, and to confide in all persons; to adopt the opinions and
habits of others; has no originality, but follows and imitates man; and
she cannot live happily without attachments, and these are sincere and
lasting, even when deserved no longer; though, from her variability of
emotion, she often quarrels temporarily with those she loves the
most;—*Varium et mutabile semper fœmina*, from the rapid change of
her emotions, is a true character; but nothing is too irksome, too
painful, or too perilous, for a mother, a wife, or a mistress, to endure
or attempt for the object of her love.[13]

For Elliotson biological difference categorically determines
gender traits. We shall see, in what follows, that the simple categorization of character attributes by sexual difference is variously reinforced and challenged in the fiction of mid-century
novelists. Brontë unsettles the conventional configuration of
female nature explicitly through Caroline's continual self-questioning, thus rendering medical explanations of female distress

---

[12] For a detailed study of Dickens's relationship with Elliotson, see Fred Kaplan, *Dickens and Mesmerism: The Hidden Springs of Fiction* (Princeton, NJ: Princeton University Press, 1975).

[13] John Elliotson, *Human Physiology*, p. 705.

uncertain and unreliable. Both the nature of Caroline's illness and the supposition of her cure are left open to conjecture. What Brontë's novel throws into relief is that the science of gender relation and differentiation is not necessarily to be trusted. For her, it is not the nature of woman that is the problem, but the assumptions which underpin and perpetuate the notion of her inherent weakness. Not just in *Shirley* but throughout Charlotte Brontë's work we are made acutely aware of the discrepancy between a woman's subjective experience of illness or distress and the objective interpretations and designations put upon it.

But the essentializing process runs deeper than the simple separation of character traits into male and female categories for the purposes of interpreting symptoms of functional disease. The gendering of concepts and values which clearly have no inherent sexual property is rooted in the pervasive Nature/Culture binary, a dichotomous mindset which, as Ludmilla Jordanova has shown, has shaped Western thought around constructs of sexual polarity.[14] Importantly, this Nature/Culture dichotomy operates paradigmatically in the literary texts and works to subsume a seemingly limitless range of disparities into an apparent system of opposites. Although the polarities of the binary are not in themselves inherently positive or negative, value and rank are ascribed to them in order to invoke a particular set of images and associations. Organizing arbitrary concepts into convenient patterns inevitably imparts a false sense of coherence and relation. Models of 'space' and 'time' and qualities such as 'active' and 'affective' were routinely gender inflected in mid-nineteenth-century formulations of health and disease. Consciously or unconsciously, writers across the disciplines make use of the multiple binaries of the interiorized/exteriorized, cyclical/linear, affective/active lives of woman/man in the representation of nervous disease and of its social meanings.[15]

One important factor in the interdisciplinary exchanges was

[14] Ludmilla Jordanova, *Sexual Visions: Images of Gender in Science and Medicine Between the Eighteenth and Twentieth Centuries* (Hemel Hempstead: Harvester Wheatsheaf, 1989).

[15] Jordanova cites G. Lloyd, *The Man of Reason: 'Male' and 'Female' in Western Philosophy* (London, 1984) for a useful philosophical debate on this subject.

the flow of ideas throughout Europe. Educated people were more likely to be literate in several European languages and, in the medical field, a British doctor's training often included long periods of study or of practice abroad, most often in France or Germany.[16] Effectively this meant that, despite national differences, cultural assumptions in respect of the gendering and hierarchizing of sickness and social role were demonstrably transportable. Daniel Pick has highlighted the European dimension by tracing ideas about 'degeneration' through France, Italy, and England, and has shown how significantly the transmission of ideas influences and modifies the cultural assumptions, politics, and language of discourse across national and disciplinary boundaries.[17] The same metaphors and paradigms into which complex concepts were over-simplified were worked into representations of disease and health, masculinity and femininity, where they held powerful sway over beliefs and attitudes far beyond national boundaries. Dickens published reviews in *Household Words* of a number of works by the French cultural historian Jules Michelet whose ideas of gendered space are revealing.[18] His blending of the mythical and the biological to justify separate spheres gives a sense of the rhetorical power of images to fix cultural attitudes. Furthermore, it exemplifies the ease with which the factors of biological sex, gender, and sickness came to be so inextricably

[16] A book which highlights the fluency of medical ideas across European countries particularly during the eighteenth and nineteenth centuries is Edward Shorter's *From Paralysis to Fatigue: A History of Psychosomatic Illness in the Modern Era* (New York: Free Press, 1992).

[17] Daniel Pick, *Faces of Degeneration: A European Disorder, c.1848—c.1918* (Cambridge: Cambridge University Press, 1989).

[18] A review of Michelet's *L'Amour* (1858) appeared on 2 April 1859, pp. 426–32. In the same year, Dickens also published reviews of *L'Insecte* and *L'Oiseau* by the same reviewer, Edmund Saul Dixon. As further evidence of the currency of Michelet's ideas in England, an anonymous article in *Blackwood's Magazine*, 86 (1859) devotes several columns to a discussion of a new book 'which has emanated from the pen of M. Michelet . . . simply entitled *L'Amour*', pp. 90–5. More generally, Michelet's book *Du prêtre, de la femme, de la famille* was translated into English by C. Cocks in the same year (1845) as its publication in France. According to Cocks, the translation sold 'fifty thousand copies into every corner of the kingdom', where it 'cannot fail to be a source of interest and edification to the greater part of my fellow-countrymen'. *Priests, Women, and Families*, trans. by C. Cocks (London: Longman, Brown, Green, and Longmans, 1845), Preface, p. xi. In the 1850s, this work was subsequently translated by G. H. Smith for Whitaker's Popular Library. By contrast, *La Femme* was not translated as far as I can establish.

intertwined and absorbed imperceptibly into medical and fictional representations of the female invalid.

Michelet's vision of essential difference crystallizes a ubiquitous paradigm according to which women's lives are perceived as cyclical and enclosed and men's as linear and progressive:

Lui, il marche de drame en drame, dont pas un ne ressemble à l'autre, d'experience en experience, et de bataille en bataille. L'Histoire va s'allonger toujours . . . et lui dit toujours . . . 'En avant!'

Elle, au contraire, elle suit la noble et sereine épopée que la Nature accompli dans ses cycles harmoniques, revenant sur elle-même, avec une grace touchante de constance et de la fidélité. Ces retours, dans son mouvement, mettent la paix, et, si j'osais dire, une immobilité relative.[19]

Despite the positive resonances in the language of cycle, harmony, constancy, and fidelity, there is a troubling sense of treadmill-like repetition. In her harmony, woman is also trapped. Cycle and enclosure here define and confine the lives of woman. Her 'cycles harmoniques' link woman in metaphorical commune with nature and in a 'noble', 'serene', and, intriguingly, 'epic' series of returns and renewals. But, by the same token, they define her as imprisoned by her own biological functioning. In the earlier *L'Amour*, Michelet had wanted it to be understood that the mysterious rhythms which characterized woman's nature also ensured a lifelong pathology in which '(one could say almost perpetually) woman is not only ill but wounded'.[20] The very language asserts that the normal process of menstruation was the sign of woman's inherently pathological state but, here again, the representation of the natural invalid is dependent upon an interweaving of metaphorical and literal sense. Unable, then, to transcend her femininity, woman is confined by her body to her cell of domesticity. The models of dynamic difference fit with, and in many ways corroborate, the gendered designations of neurosis. Where men's disease, as I shall be arguing in the next chapter, was far more likely to be regarded as a disruption, an interruption in normal healthy progress, women were held to be locked in a constant round of

[19] Jules Michelet, *La Femme* (1859), Préface de Thérèse Moreau (Paris: Flammarion, 1981), p. 148.
[20] Quoted by Ludmilla Jordanova in *Sexual Visions*, p. 79.

chronic sickness marked out by menstruation, childbirth, lactation, and the climacteric.

Examples from British doctors who devoted entire books to the pathology and treatment of the menstrual cycle alone, quite apart from the business of childbirth, are legion.[21] The idea of the female body as a cell of sickness persisted with a tenacity which seems extraordinary when placed alongside the profound treatises written by the same doctors in other areas of neurophysiology. In the last quarter of the century, Henry Maudsley was still insisting that a woman's reproductive cycle was a lifelong tyranny which, for 'the best years of life' renders her 'more or less sick and unfit for hard work'.[22] Behind this prejudice lay a great deal of ignorance and the idea of women as permanent invalids did not escape ridicule, perhaps most famously by Elizabeth Garrett Anderson in her 'Reply' to Maudsley's paper.[23] A year earlier, another woman writer had expressed her 'disgust' upon opening a recently published American book to find 'the same idea which Michelet has so sentimentally elaborated—namely, that woman's natural state is that of invalidism, and that all her peculiar natural functions' measure out her life in epochs of pain, sickness, and suffering.[24] Her mention of Michelet is an indication of the currency of his ideas in Europe and beyond even through to the latter decades of the century. Thus, when the Leeds physician Clifford Allbutt addressed the

---

[21] To mention just a few: Thomas Addison, *Observations on the Disorders of Females Connected with Uterine Irritation* (London: S. Highley, 1830); E. J. Tilt, *On the Preservation of the Health of Women at the Critical Periods of Life* (London: John Churchill, 1851); and Tilt, *On Diseases of Women and Ovarian Inflammation, in Relation to Morbid Menstruation, Sterility, Pelvic Tumours, & Affections of the Womb*, 2nd edn. (London: John Churchill, 1853); Samuel Mason, *The Philosophy of Female Health: Being an Enquiry Into Its Connection With, and Dependence Upon the Due Performance of the Uterine Functions; With Observations on the Nature, Causes, and Treatment of Female Disorders in General* (London: H. Hughes, 1845); E. H. Ruddock, *The Affections of Females, Including the Derangements Incident on Menstruation, and their Homeopathic and General Treatment* (London: Homeopathic Publishing Co., 1861).
[22] 'Sex in Mind and in Education', *Fortnightly Review*, n.s. 15 (April, 1874), 466–83 (p. 480).
[23] 'Sex in Mind and Education: A Reply', *Fortnightly Review*, n.s. 15 (May, 1874), 582–94.
[24] Eliza B. Duffey, *What Women Should Know: A Woman's Book About Women. Containing Practical Information for Wives and Mothers* (Philadelphia: [n.pub.], 1873), pp. 43–4.

medical audience of the Gulstonian Lecture in 1884, he announced that the time had surely come when that well-known 'proverb, *L'utérus c'est la femme*', should be newly examined in the more sober light of psychosomatic medicine.[25]

In different ways, and for different reasons, Brontë and Dickens engage in these debates as they explore the dynamics of sexual role and social and moral responsibility within the domestic economy. When Brontë compares Caroline's vision of the outside world of nature as 'an enchanted region' to the 'narrow chamber' of her inner experience, she speaks as much of women in general as of Caroline's particular sense of self (173). Brontë's exposure of the actual, as opposed to the idealized, female space makes explicit what Michelet's generalizations hide, namely that the seemingly benign female enclosure can also be a cell, potentially a scene of entrapment and imprisonment. *Little Dorrit*, as many critics have pointed out, is a novel of mental prisons as much as literal ones. Dickens makes the point when describing Mrs Clennam gazing down into the prison yard. 'She stood at the window', the narrator observes, 'bewildered, looking down into this prison as it were out of her own different prison'.[26] Mrs Clennam's prison of sickness is, in two senses, a close confinement. Her house is made a place of correction and quarantine where, in her role as moral agent, she seeks to eliminate the sexual taint of Arthur's illegitimate birth by preventing the transmission of its knowledge into the world beyond the house walls. Furthermore, she herself embodies, in her immobility, the extreme end of this 'close confinement' of female sensibility to the pain of disappointed expectations which Brontë depicts in poignant physical images of mental suffering and silent endurance. Literary interpretations of gendered spaces undermine not only any clear delineation between an internal world that is female and cyclical, and an external one that is male and progressive, but more importantly the positive and negative values that attach to them. Time and again, the idea of an enclosed female space as both benign and

---

[25] Allbutt's lectures are published as *On Visceral Neuroses* (London: John Churchill, 1884). See especially p. 15.

[26] Charles Dickens, *Little Dorrit* (1855–7), ed. by Stephen Wall and Helen Small (Harmondsworth: Penguin, 1998), p. 753. Subsequent references to this edition will be given in the text.

unhealthy is developed through a shared vocabulary of 'narrow' worlds. Mrs Clennam has confined herself within 'narrow limits' (185) and views the world through 'two narrow windows' (180). Caroline Helstone, as I have noted above, returns to the 'narrow chamber' of woman's social and emotional constraints. The old maids in *Shirley* are depicted in narrow circumstances which are both material and emotional, but the very sparseness of their lives confers a nun-like serenity upon their privations. The word 'narrow', and the cognate images of self-effacement and restraint, inscribe woman's domestic role in a metaphoric affinity with representations of nuns' cells, celibacy, refusal, self-denial, lack of sexual fulfilment, sorrow, loss, and religious zeal, all of which connote a rigorous subordination of sexual and sensual energies to more cerebral or spiritual obligations.

If, as I am suggesting, the gendered concepts of time and space, and of active and affective qualities, are simply absorbed as givens in the writings of medical men and social commentators, the categorization of female conformity with well-being and of transgression with disease has a simple, but convenient, logic. The idealized image of the 'angel in the house' gave rise to numerous variations on the enclosed space, the inner sanctum which both preserved woman's moral purity and ensured her dedication to her appointed task of service and humility. It was Michelet's vision of Woman in her temple within a garden that prompted Bram Dijkstra to describe her as '[s]itting in her cell outside of history, buoyed by her "relative changelessness" '.[27] Women who did not aspire to such a high calling, or who, to recall Elliotson's phrase, chose to live 'without attachments', or who were simply overlooked in the marriage markets, were generally regarded not just as a social problem but as a sexual anomaly which only the physician was qualified to interpret. However medical spokesmen justified their concerns about 'old maids', their obsession with the physical condition of the body underlines once again the importance that was placed upon the supposed link between social and sexual participation and

---

[27] Bram Dijkstra, *Idols of Perversity: Fantasies of Feminine Evil in Fin-de-Siècle Culture* (New York: Oxford University Press, 1986), p. 12.

physiological health.[28] Charlotte Brontë merely reproduces the standard rhetoric on old maids when, on the occasion of her visit to Miss Mann and Miss Ainley, Caroline Helstone notes with dread for her own future the ruinous effects upon the body of a life presumed to be emotionally and sexually arid. From a male standpoint, the generally held view is that of Robert Moore, who habitually compares Caroline's 'fair youth—delicate and attractive' with the withered body of the 'shrivelled eld, livid and loveless', whose conversation had soured into 'the vinegar discourse of a cankered old maid' (177). Caroline's resolve to avoid such a fate implicitly strengthens the conceptual model of the morbid registration upon the body of self-denial, sacrifice, and lack. In psychosomatic terms, mental, emotional, and intellectual starvation are translated into bodily atrophy.

At the same time that doctors were emphasizing the morbid consequences to female health of an unfulfilled sexual life, others were busy denying that women had 'sexual feeling of any kind'.[29] William Acton's much-quoted pronouncements were attempts to justify woman's suitability for her roles of moral superintendent and domestic angel. With a few sad exceptions, writes Acton, 'there can be no doubt that sexual feeling in the female is in the majority of cases in abeyance, and that it requires positive and considerable excitement to be roused at all'.[30] Although Acton was not highly regarded amid medical circles, where he was more of a self-publicist than a luminary, the premiss that women were fitted, by virtue of their natural passionlessness, even frigidity, for the role of moral guardian, gave rise to many tenuous representations of Victorian womanhood. Apart from the obvious contradiction in a theory which claims simultaneously, on behalf of women, that sexual desire is non-existent, and that it is latent but kept in abeyance, Acton's

---

[28] On the 'Old Maids' debate, see Anon., 'Woman in Her Psychological Relations', (n. 10 above), pp. 34–6; W. R. Greg, 'Why are Women Redundant?', *National Review*, 14 (1862), 434–60; Frances Power Cobbe, 'What Shall We Do with Our Old Maids?', *Fraser's Magazine*, 66 (1862), 594–610; W. G. Hamley, 'Old Maids', *Blackwood's Magazine*, 112 (1872), 94-108.

[29] William Acton, *The Functions and Disorders of the Reproductive Organs in Childhood, in Youth, in Adult Age, and in Advanced Life, Considered in Their Physiological, Social and Moral Relations*, 4th edn. (London: John Churchill, 1865), p. 112.

[30] *The Functions and Disorders*, p. 112.

theory of sexual difference slips, it seems, between essence and degree.[31] The difficulty medical spokesmen faced was the need to square the idea of woman as wife and mother with the ideal of moral purity and it was hardly surprising that their convoluted efforts produced contradictory pictures. Their attempts to explain female sexuality, however nonsensical they now seem, or indeed seemed at the time, are important in bringing to the fore the knot of dilemmas with which both doctors and their female patients had to wrestle. Of these, one of the most troublesome was the contradiction between the scientifically sanctioned view of woman as mentally inferior—the child-woman, passive, fragile, nervously susceptible, who needed a husband to supply the qualities she so obviously lacked—and the culturally sustained view of the 'angel' whose natural moral sovereignty appointed her to maintain domestic harmony and to keep her husband from undue excess.

Charlotte Brontë is much clearer than Acton seems to be on the matter of a discrepancy between female sexuality and the gendered assumptions drawn from its inexpressibility. Seeking to unpick the idealized notions of womanhood which hinder expression of the subjective and the 'real', Brontë's portrayal of Caroline Helstone's dilemma tacitly poses the question: how is it possible to express female feelings, as opposed to feminine virtues, in a positive way? John Maynard has argued that Brontë's overriding concern is 'for values that are not sexual within her general concern with sexual maturation'.[32] While this may be partly true, I think it falls short of the point. Her concern is rather for positive value in sexuality. What Caroline is offered instead are images of maturation, of love, and of

[31] Like W. R.Greg before him, and from whom he quotes, Acton's tendentious assertions were prompted by the need to resolve contradictions in Victorian sexual ideology for which they themselves, as self-appointed experts on moral and social matters, were partly responsible. For a full discussion of the inconsistencies inherent in Victorian pronouncements on female sexuality which seek to distinguish between classes of women whilst, at the same time, representing all women as 'essentially asexual, self-sacrificing, and passive', see Mary Poovey, 'Speaking of the Body: Mid-Victorian Constructions of Female Desire', in Mary Jacobus, Evelyn Fox Keller, and Sally Shuttleworth (eds.), *Body/Politics: Women and the Discourses of Science* (New York: Routledge, 1990), pp. 29–46.

[32] John Maynard, *Charlotte Brontë and Sexuality* (Cambridge: Cambridge University Press, 1984), pp. 155–6.

marriage that, far from enabling expression of sexuality, work to stifle and suppress it. Fantasies of love, fed by a diet of romantic literature, are all 'false pictures', warns Mrs Pryor, and must be abandoned if a woman is wise. 'They are not like reality: they show you only the green tempting surface of the marsh, and give not one faithful or truthful hint of the slough underneath' (379).[33] Immured in ignorance and constrained by a code of self-effacement, resistance to the essentializing assumptions about women's nature is made impossible in a culture which proscribes self-expression.

For Caroline Helstone, the problem consists in an incongruity of values and desires. Forced to confront the contradictions between social expectation and her own needs, she agonizes over the inequity of a world in which one sex is assumed to be more 'naturally' fitted to self-sacrifice:

Where is my place in the world? . . . Your place is to do good to others, to be helpful whenever help is wanted. That is right in some measure, and a very convenient doctrine for the people who hold it; but I perceive that certain sets of human beings are very apt to maintain that other sets should give up their lives to them and their service, and then they requite them by praise: they call them devoted and virtuous. Is this enough? Is it to live? Is there not a terrible hollowness, mockery, want, craving, in that existence which is given away to others, for want of something of your own to bestow it on? I suspect there is. Does virtue lie in abnegation of self? I do not believe it. Undue humility makes tyranny; weak concession creates selfishness. (174)

The immediate reason for Caroline's distress is Robert Moore's lack of interest in her and the prospect, as she sees it, of becoming an old maid. There are difficulties for a modern reader with a heroine for whom marriage and motherhood are the supreme attainments. But the interrogative impulse of this outburst

---

[33] Many medical texts are scathing about romantic literature and cite novels in particular as responsible for over-stimulating the imagination, thereby causing hallucination, delusion, loss of a grip on reality, and nervous disease. Contrastingly, French novels were condemned by medical critics for presenting a dangerously realistic picture of life. In *Shirley*, Mr Sympson voices his alarm when Shirley Keeldar describes a satisfactory marriage as one in which a wife is free to do as she pleases: 'You read French. Your mind is poisoned with French novels. You have imbibed French principles' (p. 550). 'French principles' was a term used more widely to describe critical attitudes towards political or religious authority; it stemmed, no doubt, from Revolutionary ideas.

discloses a scepticism on the part of Brontë about the institutionalized structures which define and limit woman's choices.
Caroline's tormented self-questioning as to the value of a life of
selfless devotion to others mounts a bold challenge to the
rubrics of female conduct laid down in contemporary middle-
class advice books. Indeed, she voices that which writers like
Sarah Stickney Ellis began ironically to hint at, namely the
wastefulness of empty sacrifice.[34] More broadly, the rhetorical
cast of some of her questions exposes a real futility behind all
the heroic rhetoric of ideal womanhood.

DISAPPOINTMENT AND DECLINE:
SHIRLEY, ADELA CATHCART, DEERBROOK

When, during a reading of *Coriolanus* at the Moore household,
Caroline attempts to awaken Robert Moore to 'feelings' which
she believes have been suppressed by a masculine education, a
narratorial observation seems to confirm her nature, not his
emotional reticence as problematic. A quality in her manner
that evening is described by the narrator in terms which echo
John Elliotson's analysis of woman's 'variability' and 'rapid
change' of emotion:

It may be remarked, in passing, that the general character of her
conversation that evening, whether serious or sprightly, grave or gay,
was as of something untaught, unstudied, intuitive, fitful; when once
gone, no more to be reproduced as it had been, than the glancing ray
of the meteor, than the tints of the dew-gem, than the colour or form
of the sun-set cloud, than the fleeting and glittering ripple varying the
flow of a rivulet. (91)

Caroline's endeavour to dissolve rigid gender difference into
complementarity collapses in constructions of the female body

---

34 When Ellis wrote, for instance, that a woman's world was 'one where pleasure
of the highest, purest order, naturally and necessarily arises out of acts of duty faith-
fully performed', or that woman 'is never more truly great than when willingly and
judiciously performing kind offices for the sick', she is advocating not so much that
women accept these tenets *per se* but that they might usefully turn a requirement
into a reason for better education in the knowledge and skills necessary to fulfil it.
See *The Women of England: Their Social Duties and Domestic Habits* (London:
Fisher, 1838), pp. 19, 41.

as unstable, female nature as mutable and impermanent. Throughout the novel, the fluctuations in Caroline's bodily state are, in obvious ways, related to her emotional state but, more complexly, to her anxiousness to fathom why female feelings constitute such a problem for social stability in the first place.

Medical men were in little doubt that woman's greater sensitivity to emotion made her less capable of controlling her will and, therefore, more prone to nervous disease. Robert Brudenell Carter explained how women were doubly disadvantaged, first by nature and then by social injunction. Writing in 1853, Carter affirms that susceptibility to hysterical outbursts is 'considerably greater in the woman than in the man, partly from that *natural* conformation which causes the former to feel, under circumstances where the latter thinks; and partly because the woman is more often under the necessity of endeavouring to conceal her feelings'.[35] The questionable logic which holds that, on the one hand, women are emotionally fitful, weak and vulnerable and, on the other, capable of astonishing endurance—we may recall Elliotson's observation that 'nothing is too irksome, too painful, or too perilous, for a mother, a wife, or a mistress, to endure or attempt for the object of her love'— forces Brontë to a powerful articulation of the deadlock into which severe social prescriptions have placed women. To labour constantly with the incompatibilities between private experience and social circumscription is, as Terry Eagleton has commented, to live with the lie of ever having to conceal 'private agony' behind a 'public mask'.[36] Brontë inveighs against the 'public mask' in images of profound physical pain:

Take the matter as you find it: ask no questions; utter no remonstrances: it is your best wisdom. You expected bread, and you have got a stone; break your teeth on it, and don't shriek because the nerves are martyrized: do not doubt that your mental stomach—if you have such a thing—is strong as an ostrich's—the stone will digest. You held out your hand for an egg, and fate put into it a scorpion. Show no consternation: close your fingers firmly upon the gift; let it sting through your palm. Never mind: in time, after your hand and arm have swelled and

[35] Robert Brudenell Carter, *On the Pathology and Treatment of Hysteria* (London: John Churchill, 1853), p. 33.
[36] Terry Eagleton, *Myths of Power: A Marxist Study of the Brontës* (London: Macmillan, 1975), p. 57.

quivered long with torture, the squeezed scorpion will die, and you will have learned the great lesson how to endure without a sob. For the whole remnant of your life, if you survive the test—some, it is said, die under it—you will be stronger, wiser, less sensitive. (105)

The central image of the 'mental stomach' encapsulates the internalization by women of the social and medical edicts (figured in the ingestion and (in)digestion of foreign matter) until no trace of the pain and suffering they cause is visible on the outside. Among women writers, such images were evocative of the strength of the social conventions which restricted expressions of passion to the pages of fiction. Harriet Martineau, whose highly reputed political and social writings Charlotte Brontë is known to have admired, wrote only one novel, *Deerbrook*. Published in 1839, and recalled in her *Autobiography* as having been written as 'a relief to many pent-up sufferings, feelings and convictions', the book contains a passage which is strikingly similar to the one above.[37]

During a discussion between two women friends, Maria, a governess whose succession of illnesses have left her a cripple, speaks of the agony of a woman's silent endurance of the passion of love which has nothing to do with marriage, and which 'shakes her being to the very centre—more awful, more tremendous, than the crack of doom':

'But why? Why so tremendous?'
'From the struggle which it calls upon her to endure, silently and alone;—from the agony of a change of existence which must be wrought without any eye perceiving it. ... Our being can but be strained till not another effort can be made. This is all that we can conceive to happen in death; and it happens in love, with the additional burden of fearful secresy. One may lie down and await death, with sympathy about one to the last, though the passage hence must be solitary; and it would be a small trouble if all the world looked on to see the parting of soul and body: but that other passage into a new state, that other process of becoming a new creature, must go on in the darkness of the spirit, while the body is up and abroad, and no one must know what is passing within. The spirit's leap from heaven to hell must be made while the smile is on the lips, and light words are upon

[37] *Harriet Martineau's Autobiography*, vol. 2 (1877), p. 113, quoted in Harriet Martineau, *Deerbrook* (1839), with intro. by Gaby Weiner (New York: The Dial Press, 1983), p. vii.

the tongue. The struggles of shame, the pangs of despair, must be hidden in the depths of the prison-house. Every groan must be stifled before it is heard: and as for tears—they are a solace too gentle for the case. The agony is too strong for tears'.[38]

Maria's companion, Margaret, listens with growing dismay to the unending sufferings which await the woman in love. Casting aside the traditional notion of the weaker sex, Maria ascribes women's exceptional fortitude to the 'power of self-restraint . . . under which we all lie'. And ten years before Caroline Helstone bravely challenged the system of values which expects self-sacrifice from one sex and not the other, Martineau's Maria doubts that the pain of self-restraint ever bestowed nobility. We have to believe, she continues, that some 'moral and intellectual good—must issue from such exercise and discipline as this' otherwise the crazed brains, crippled bodies, disease, and death that such mental suffering produces will amount to nothing in the progression towards a more enlightened society.[39] The difficulty, however, of promoting a life of honest expression within a marriage hidebound by convention is one Margaret faces when she is torn between sisterly sympathy with the unhappily married Hester and her perceived duty to support Hester's husband, the doctor Mr Hope. In what seems almost a betrayal of Maria's persuasions, Margaret steels herself against Hester's despair and agrees with Hope that hysterical outbursts are not to be tolerated. With their help, emotional 'sluices' will be kept firmly shut and Hester must learn how to act.[40] Although the marriage is as miserable for Hope as it is for Hester, Martineau makes it clear that, while the husband will seek solace in his work, the wife must somehow find reserves of strength within herself in order to present an outward appearance of solidity to the world.

As medical science pursued the hypothesis that mental and moral attributes and deficiencies were discernible in the physical appearance of the body, notions of body legibility filtered down into the popular imagination through the marginal sciences of physiognomy and phrenology.[41] With advocates

---

[38] *Deerbrook*, pp. 159–60.   [39] Ibid., pp. 163–4.
[40] Ibid., p. 208.
[41] The theory of phrenology was formulated at the end of the eighteenth century by the Viennese physician Franz Joseph Gall. Developing hand in hand with the science of cerebral localization, it was made popular in Britain by George Combe.

among eminent physicians and alienists, phrenology lent plausibility to the perception of the body as a sign, an indicator, not only of inner psychological make-up, but of an individual's conformity to, or deviation from, dominant social and moral codes. On principles which have already been set out, the signs of normative (and healthy) femininity were, somewhat paradoxically, sought in self-effacement and passivity. Whether the woman's body outwardly reflected a husband's or family's social status, or became a mere register of something that is projected onto it through the desires, fantasies, or idealizations of others, the virtues of self-effacement and passivity were satisfactorily demonstrated.[42] By contrast, deviation was reflected in agency. Thus, the female body which articulated its own physical and emotional needs through visible symptoms was one which was sick. But further twists of logic serve to sanction the sick body as a permissible sign of female selfhood, inasmuch as infirmity accords with the constructions of woman's natural weakness and vulnerability.

Under these kinds of constraints, Caroline Helstone is driven to hide herself away from prying and 'reading' eyes as she grows ill with pining from unrequited love. Languishing under the pressure of the strength of her feelings of desire and loss, and yet ever under the injunction to conceal them, Caroline's dread is that her body will betray her; that, by its appearance, its attitude, movements, and gestures, it will make visible to an inquisitive audience its drama of sexual awakening. Aware of the necessity of self-regulation, she kept 'her pale face and wasted figure as much out of sight as she could' in order to allay the curiosity of 'young ladies [who] looked at her in a way she understood, and from whom she shrank', as well as the speculation of old ladies who 'were always offering her their advice,

For analyses of the rise and popularity of the science of phrenology in Britain, see Robert M. Young, *Mind, Brain and Adaptation in the Nineteenth Century* (Oxford: Clarendon Press, 1970); Roger Cooter, *The Cultural Meaning of Popular Science: Phrenology and the Organization of Consent in Nineteenth-Century Britain* (Cambridge: Cambridge University Press, 1984); Sally Shuttleworth, *Charlotte Brontë and Victorian Psychology* (Cambridge: Cambridge University Press, 1996), chapter 4.

[42] For a fuller discussion of the reading of moral states on the body, see Lynda Nead, *Myths of Sexuality: Representations of Women in Victorian Britain* (Oxford: Blackwell, 1988), p. 170.

recommending this or that nostrum' (192). Brontë's narrative of Caroline's decline into love-sickness draws on standard images of the wilting romantic heroine. When we read of how, in her 'utter sickness of longing and disappointment' over her rejection by Robert, Caroline succumbs to a vague and indefinable debility characterized by loss of flesh and vitality, it is impossible not to be struck by the resonances of fading Ophelias in sentimentalized portrayals of female repressed desire. An association between the acute disappointment of love and stifled sexual expression accounts for a proliferation of images, in art and in literature, of pining, wasting women with self-consuming sicknesses. Some of these images take the form of idealizations born of male fantasies, as in the pre-Raphaelite paintings and poetry depicting courtly ladies and mythical Venuses translated into Victorian contexts of madness and death.[43] Of Caroline Helstone, we are told that she had changed, that 'the rose had dwindled and faded to a mere snowdrop: bloom had vanished, flesh wasted; she sat before [her uncle] drooping, colourless and thin' (189). But although Brontë clearly exploits the familiarity of these images, she does not present them uncritically.

Her representation of Caroline's ailing health as love-sickness is conscious of its own fictionality. It is the plain-speaking Mrs Yorke, who, though ridiculing Caroline's sorrowful features, brings us closer to Brontë's sense of the impossible dilemma of female suffering and its inexpressibility:

'You *feel*! Yes! yes! I daresay, now: you are led a great deal by your *feelings*, and you think yourself a very sensitive, refined personage, no doubt. Are you aware that, with all these romantic ideas, you have managed to train your features into an habitually lackadaisical expression, better suited to a novel-heroine than to a woman who is to make her way in the real world, by dint of common sense?'   (402, emphasis in original)

Mrs Yorke's deep distrust of 'feelings' and her antipathy to the 'shrinking, sensitive . . . nervous temperament' (404) make the link between pent-up desire and the languid, exhausted demeanour which was reproduced in images of collapsing

---

[43] For a study of the production and consumption of pre-Raphaelite images of women, see Lynne Pearce, *Woman, Image, Text: Readings in Pre-Raphaelite Art and Literature* (Hemel Hempstead: Harvester Wheatsheaf, 1991).

women in nineteenth-century art and in medical representation.[44] Although Caroline's chronic debility takes its form and
expression from the cultural association of the pining of unrequited love and the cachexia (extreme wasting, emaciation) of
the body, it is allied by Brontë to contemporary medical models
of the mental causes of physical disease.[45]

Disappointments, unfulfilled hopes, and unrequited love are
frequently cited by doctors among the causes of hysteria. John
Conolly advises practitioners to look to circumstantial causes
and take heed of such diagnostic signs as 'the disappointments
of females who begin to feel that they are no longer young, and
yet who have not become wives'. In a country, he adds, 'where
the passions and emotions have but a limited external manifestation, and where the female character is less intensely
expressed', practitioners 'sometimes seem to forget their silent
operation on the frame'.[46] The psychosomatic potential of
'disappointment' to weaken the whole constitution was also
recognized. James Clark documented the association between
female love-longing and the wasting symptoms (phthisis) of
consumptive disease. 'Mental depression', he writes, 'holds a
very conspicuous place among those circumstances which
diminish the powers of the system generally, and often proves
one of the most effectual determining causes of phthisis'.[47]
George MacDonald takes precisely this alleged clinical association between disappointment and decline in young women to
expound a doctrine of spiritual healing.

Adela Cathcart is not so much the story of the eponymous
heroine's illness as of the means and methods of bringing about
her cure. A young doctor, Henry Armstrong, is persuaded by
Colonel Cathcart to undertake the treatment of his ailing

[44] Bram Dijkstra's collection of visual representations of women in various stages
of exhaustion and collapse focuses on the last quarter of the century, but the group-
ing of the images into medical classifications is strongly suggestive of the cultural
associations I am underlining. For example: 'Raptures of Submission'; 'The Cult of
Invalidism; Ophelia and Folly; Dead Ladies and the Fetish of Sleep'; 'The Collapsing
Woman'; 'The Nymph With the Broken Back'. See *Idols of Perversity*.

[45] Conversely, medical writers were not above drawing on literary and artistic
images for their constructions of disease paradigms. See Helen Small, *Love's
Madness: Medicine, the Novel, and Female Insanity 1800–1865* (Oxford:
Clarendon Press, 1996), especially chapter 2.

[46] 'Hysteria', in *The Cyclopaedia of Practical Medicine*, ii. p. 572.

[47] 'Tubercular phthisis', in *The Cyclopaedia of Practical Medicine*, iv. p. 321.

daughter, Adela. Applying the same diagnostic criteria as that set out by Conolly and Clark, Armstrong first questions Cathcart about his daughter's emotional state and, in particular, about any disappointment she may have had. Although Cathcart replies in the negative, Armstrong pursues this line of enquiry, assuring him that such cases are common among girls of her age:

It is as if, without any disease, life were gradually withdrawn itself [*sic*]—ebbing back as it were to its source. Whether this has a physical or a psychological cause, it is impossible to tell. In her case, I think the later, if indeed it have not a deeper cause; that is, if I'm right in my hypothesis. A few days will show me this; and if I am wrong, I will then make a closer examination of her case. At present it is desirable that I should not annoy her in any such way. Now for the practical: my conviction is that the best thing that can be done for her is, to interest her in something, if possible—no matter what it is. Does she take pleasure in anything?[48]

On the basis of Armstrong's belief that the cause of Adela's depressive illness is a spiritual starvation from which she has lost the will to seek relief, John Smith (the narrator), Cathcart, and Armstrong together devise a programme of storytelling and music to encourage 'the tide of life [to] begin to flow again' (51). It is one of the conditions of the treatment that the invalid should remain ignorant of the male 'conspiracy' to restore her to social and psychological normality.

One of the interesting parallels with Brontë's depiction of invalidism is MacDonald's use of alimentary paradigms to examine the connections between bodily and mental illness. Brontë's image of the mental stomach where painful experiences are ingested and assimilated away from outside observation is echoed in the not unsympathetic medical view expressed by Armstrong that women may 'go into a consumption' on account of the miserable diet offered them at the 'Father's table'; a diet consisting of no more than the dry husks left over after the men have taken their nourishment (52). Furthermore, just as Caroline Helstone's hungry imagination and intellectual curiosity are ill nourished by the fantasies of love in romantic fiction

[48] George MacDonald, *Adela Cathcart* (1864) (Whitethorn, Calif.: Johannesen, 1994), p. 50.

for women, so Adela Cathcart's mind has been 'fed upon slops'. Little wonder, remarks Armstrong, that 'an atrophy is the consequence' (52). Through the narrator, John Smith, MacDonald develops the argument for the need of moral and spiritual sustenance to strengthen both body and mind:

Now from whatever cause, Adela is in a kind of moral atrophy, for she cannot digest the food provided for her, so as to get any good of it. Suppose a patient in a corresponding physical condition, should show a relish for anything proposed to him, would you not take it for a sign that that was just the thing to do him good? And we may accept the interest Adela shows in any kind of mental pabulum provided for her, as an analogous sign. It corresponds to relish, and is a ground for expecting some benefit to follow—in a word, some nourishment of the spiritual life.   (110)

Knowing that emotions had the power to lay the body low, it seemed self-evident that reviving the spirits was the best remedy for the body's state of decline. Not that this is sufficient in itself, but rather that, as John Smith remarks, first drawing the patient out of her morbid self-obsession will 'give a fair chance' to medicaments which 'act most rapidly on a system in movement' (51). From the strictly medical point of view, the effect of emotional causes is to depress the nervous constitution, thus rendering the body more susceptible to physical disease: this mechanism is one examined by Charlotte Brontë.

When Brontë aligns Caroline's burgeoning sexuality with her disappointment in love, and with the necessity to conceal both her desire and her loss, her terms of reference precisely echo medical descriptions of the combined effect of emotional and cultural agencies acting upon the body in susceptible constitutions:

She was now precisely in that state, when, if her constitution had contained the seeds of consumption, decline or slow fever, those diseases would have been rapidly developed, and would soon have carried her quietly from the world. People never die of love or grief alone; though some die of inherent maladies, which the tortures of those passions prematurely force into destructive action.   (191)

Caroline's sexual awakening proceeds in parallel with her gradual decline into illness. But, although she 'wasted, grew more joyless and more wan' as her mind 'kept harping on the name of Robert Moore' (184), it is not until she is exposed to the pathogens believed to be carried in miasma, or poisoned air, that her nebulous malady develops into the more clinically recognizable disease of brain fever.

Acceptance of the prognosis that Caroline is unlikely to die of her sorrow raises the question of the somatic reality of her illness. That question is implicit, it seems to me, in the narratorial suggestions that Caroline is consciously playing a role; the role of the consumptive romantic heroine. At first, Caroline attempts to assuage her sorrow by sublimating its intensities into good works. But the mind's concentration upon denial of the body's hunger only sustains attention upon it and prolongs the very pain and grief it seeks to disperse. One of the well-documented observations of the symptoms of hysteria, a disease known for its imitation of morbid organic states, was the female patient's skill in perpetuating the deception. Although Brontë does not make this suggestion explicit, there are hints at Caroline's complicity in her suffering, most notably in her ritualistic renewal of her disappointment. 'On a certain day in the week, at a certain hour', it is explained, Caroline 'suffered to sit in her chair near the window . . . whatever degree of exhaustion or debility her wan aspect betrayed' (425), refusing all entreaty, she watched and pined, returning to her sickbed weaker than ever. These hints at complicity are not, I suggest, accusatory in the manner of Mrs Yorke's remarks. Indeed, it could be argued that the proscription on expression gives the love-sick heroine no choice. If, as doctors generally agreed, illness was the natural condition of women, it is also the consequence of social constructions of femininity.

Everywhere in Brontë's text, ambiguity and nuance undermine attempts to define a consistent reading of the social meaning of female disease. If verbal expression is impermissible for women, the narrative revealed by the body is the only one available, but the integrity of that narrative is, as Brontë demonstrates, highly questionable. The reliability of physical signs to reveal the truth of silent suffering is lost in the gap of interpretation. The fear that one's emotional secrets might be read, or inadvertently given away, through body language, or worse, misread and misrepresented in the public domain, unsurprisingly led women to be ever vigilant of their bodies. The fear of hysteria or madness was as much a fear of interpretation as of disease itself.[49] Anxieties about the externalization of psychological distress only served to strengthen belief in the pathological consequences of repression. But Caroline Helstone does not go mad or die of love. In a sense, although it is an equivocal one, she is cured. Ostensibly, Mrs Pryor, Caroline's long-lost mother, nurses her back to health. But even as we read these nursing scenes, there are undercurrents which both challenge such optimistic readings and force us, time and again, to reconsider the meanings of 'cure' and 'recovery' where Caroline is concerned.

Some recent studies of Victorian medical discourse and fiction have emphasized the therapeutic aspects of affective exchange between the nurse/mother and patient/daughter. Where Athena Vrettos proportions Caroline's restoration to health to the mother's 'privileged capacities for interpreting the external signs of internal emotions', Miriam Bailin argues that it is Caroline's release to her invalidism and to Mrs Pryor's nursing care which enables the patient, formerly 'a mere shadow in the "real world" [to become] substantial again in the "enchanted region" of the sickroom'.[50] That the discovery of her identity while she is being nursed through her fever is crucial to Caroline's restoration to health, as critics acknowledge, is certainly borne out in the text. From a position of psychological alienation, social displacement, and economic superfluity, Caroline recovers both health and identity through the establishment of physical bonds. We are told that the 'loneliness and gloom' which had crushed Caroline's spirits 'were now banished from her bedside', and replaced with 'protection and solace'. 'She and her nurse', remarks the narrator, 'coalesced in wondrous union' (423–4). Reading these lines, visions of the woman's domain of spiritual harmony, nurturing, and renewal return to mind. But it seems to me that Brontë problematizes any notions of female solidarity in this text, including the idea of matriarchal bonding as a refuge from the oppressive masculine world outside.

---

[49] For a much more detailed exploration of the powerful image of the love-mad woman in shaping ideas of female insanity, see Helen Small's *Love's Madness*.

[50] *Somatic Fictions*, p. 42; Miriam Bailin, *The Sickroom in Victorian Fiction: The Art of Being Ill* (Cambridge: Cambridge University Press, 1994), p. 61.

It has been argued that representations of matriarchal affinities in female-authored nineteenth-century novels might be interpreted analogically as an emerging 'female sub-culture' within which women, though confined to their 'proper sphere of womanhood' and subordinated to the 'dominant culture', used the shared secrets and rituals of woman's physical experience to promote a kind of inner circle of 'female solidarity'.[51] While this inclusive model puts a positive twist, albeit retrospectively, on a cultural prescription, its suggestion of a continuity of experience among women writers, writers and readers, and fictional characters overstates the case for a unity of consciousness. And, indeed, in a book published three years before Showalter formulated the model in *A Literature of Their Own*, Patricia Beer had pointed out: 'We find little solidarity among middle-class women in the novels. Shirley and Caroline come closest to it, but there are strange betrayals in their friendship'.[52] Brontë's representation of the shared rituals and secret emotional truths reveals the extent of the influence of the ideological construct of gendered, hierarchized, separate spheres, but is shot through with disturbing ambiguity and unanswered questions. Far from endorsing Elliotson's medical, or Michelet's cultural, vision of woman's perfection in quiet, cloistered devotion, Brontë writes of a sequestered space which traps women in an affective cultural heritage reinforced by myth and sentiment.[53] Throughout *Shirley*, the language of narrow cells and cloistered lives, in which the choices open to women are spelled out as 'old maid' celibacy or hazardous marriage and motherhood, both of which are deleterious to health, is clear enough.

Of course, the renewal of the mother–daughter bond is instrumental in restoring Caroline's mental and bodily health. But the construction of universal ideological meanings from the nurturing female role, so smoothly executed in socio-medical texts, does not survive scrutiny in Brontë's novel. While she

---

[51] Elaine Showalter, *A Literature of Their Own: British Women Novelists From Brontë to Lessing* (Princeton, NJ: Princeton University Press, 1977), pp. 14–15.

[52] Patricia Beer, *Reader, I Married Him* (London: Macmillan, 1974), p. 118.

[53] Jules Michelet theorized a 'feminine' history as opposed to the great sweep of mainstream masculine history. He called it her *'chère légende'*, a phrase which linguistically inscribes women into a mythical cultural heritage: *'la légende'* also translates as 'inscription'. *La Femme*, p. 149.

seems close to affirming a matriarchal continuity of replenish-
ment and care, the sense of entrapment in the sickroom scene is
impossible to ignore. Momentarily, it is true, the cloistered
space of female affect 'dispels the disruptive "other"' of
doctors, husbands, and lovers.[54] Bailin rightly questions the
efficacy of the sickroom's transformative dynamic to 'inform or
revitalize the world outside its walls'.[55] But even within the
shared experience of the healing ritual, Brontë introduces
disturbing undercurrents and intrusions into the supposed cell
of solace. It is, after all, in the sickroom that Mrs Pryor relates
the harrowing details of her violent marriage to her patient,
Caroline, who is already 'crushed' and 'broken' (432) with
yearning for a romantic vision of a relationship of undying love.
Far from dispelling the 'disruptive other', it is her intervention
which introduces the male 'other' as a 'disruptive' force, thereby
modifying her daughter's understanding and exacerbating her
condition even as it seems designed to assuage it. Her explanation for abandoning the infant daughter whose pretty features
seemed to bear the 'stamp of perversity' in order to save herself,
already 'galled, crushed, paralyzed, dying' (437) from the yoke
of marriage, is hardly a palliative one. Perhaps for Mrs Pryor
the sickroom is a refuge from the tyranny of life, a retreat from
'bondage', and from the terror of a renewed 'irruption of
violence and vice!' (438). For Caroline, it works rather to
replace her girlish fantasies of a marriage of complementarity
with view of adult life as a coming to terms with unpalatable
truths of sexuality. To speak of Caroline's recovery is premature.
The therapeutic process is rather a process of adjustment during
which Brontë's youthful romantic heroine is divested of sentimentalism and integrated into a reality of disappointment.

The perpetuation through the generations of optimism in
spite of experience is something which did not escape Harriet
Martineau's critical eye. When Maria disabuses Margaret of
romantic notions of marriage, she explains how, against all the
odds, '[e]very mother and friend hopes that no one else has
suffered as she did—that her particular charge may escape
entirely, or get off more easily'. Mothers will resist confessing to
their daughters because of the shame confession brings. Some

---

[54] *The Sickroom in Victorian Fiction*, p. 64.   [55] Ibid., p. 69.

women may conclude, she adds, 'that they must have exaggerated their own sufferings, or have been singularly rebellious and unreasonable'. Brontë seems almost to dramatize what Martineau pondered in the dialogue between Margaret and Maria. 'When you remember, too, that it is the law of nature and providence that each should bear his and her own burden, and that no warning should be of any avail, it seems no longer so strange', Maria suggests, that girls 'reared in a maidenly pride, and an innocent confidence' will continue to suffer the agonies of their forebears.[56] There is a continuity, also, between Martineau's and Brontë's examination of what seems a ludicrous prohibition on female/male friendships based purely on mutual interests. The companionship of one's brother's friends, for instance, is sure to attract unwanted attention and to invite speculation of the most wounding kind. Through Maria, Martineau presents a disturbing agenda for an innocent girl's lessons in womanhood.

Brontë's writing continues to unsettle attempts to identify a formula for the relationship between female health and conformity to social role. No sooner has Caroline been apprised of the facts which seem to confirm the rigid essentialist divisions in male and female sexuality, status, and empowerment, than we find her communing in a garden with a man with whom, uniquely in her experience, she 'found plenty to talk about' (445). For Caroline, the garden and not the sickroom becomes the convalescent respite, both from the world she must ultimately re-enter and from the one she shared with her mother. In this intermediate realm, the improbable affinity between Caroline and the gardener, William Farren, quite emphatically excludes and distances the mother. Farren's 'very fine feelings' are completely at odds with Mrs Pryor's perception of the 'great gulf' which separates sexes and classes. The empathy between Caroline and Farren belies those simplistic essentialist divisions by displacing the mother, who was left 'walking near', in preference for the 'rough-handed, rough-headed, fustian-clad clown' (446) to effect the restoration of tranquillity of body and mind. Low class and male sex are radically transformed by Brontë into healing influences. But if the garden space enables

[56] *Deerbrook*, pp. 160–2.

rituals of transvaluation that seem impossible beyond its boundary walls, what figurative status does it have in the wider pattern of experience? Despite the released flow of feelings made possible by the easy reciprocity between Caroline and Farren, there seems little respite and no cure in this temporary suspension that is sustainable in the world to which the convalescent must return. When Caroline is restored to her mother's possessive guardianship, the claustrophobia is palpable. Brontë's scepticism as to the positive, ameliorative functioning of the enclosed female domain testifies to the inadequacy of the conceptual framework of gendered space.

Many feminist critiques of Victorian medicine and its treatment of women have highlighted a culture of oppression and disregarded the possibility that the overriding desire of the majority of doctors was to heal their patients. That said, it is clear from most medical reports that the practitioner's aim was to restore their female patients to their proper functioning within the domestic economy. 'Cure' did not carry connotations of a recovered sense of self-worth nor of restoration to a level of autonomy and control. The ambiguous meanings of Caroline's 'cure' and the troubling ending of the novel press the question of whether we are back where we began; namely, that the return to health is made synonymous with a return to mute compliance. When the crisis is over, Caroline is reinstated within the orthodox parameters of the dominant culture as if in a weary final capitulation to a history shaped by men. The uneasy sense of acquiescence is noted by Pauline Nestor, who writes of how, despite the novel's 'fairy-tale' conclusion of the double marriages, we are left with 'more sense of disturbance and discontent than of resolution'.[57] Brontë's palpable anxiety about the possibility of a reconciliation between the separate realms of experience registers in the incompatibility of the hopes and dreams of Robert and Caroline in respect of the wooded environs of Hollows Mill, and, even more disturbingly, in Shirley's relinquishing of her freedom. Beneath the playfulness of Shirley's coaxing of Louis Moore into adopting a suitably dominating masculine role lies a disquieting sense of the imprisoning nature of role conformity. In language which deliberately

[57] Pauline Nestor, *Charlotte Brontë* (London: Macmillan, 1983), p. 79.

blurs the boundaries between bonds and bondage, desire and enslavement, the narrator announces Shirley's forthcoming marriage as a triumph over rebellious female resistance: 'It had needed a sort of tempest-shock to bring her to the point; but there she was at last, fettered to a fixed day: there she lay, conquered by love, and bound with a vow . . . vanquished and restricted, she pined, like any other chained denizen of deserts' (637).[58]

Despite the self-conscious appeal to the romantic comedy denouement, it is the sense of 'fatigued acquiescence' which sets the tone of the ending of *Shirley*.[59] The unease noted by Nestor and others is on account of the uncertain future for Shirley and Caroline. To return for a moment to the medical and cultural-historical contexts of Brontë's writing, it would seem that the theories about woman's nature, about repression and disease, and about cyclic rather than progressive history, justify that disquiet by maintaining the inevitability of capitulation. As has been demonstrated, the defining characteristics of Victorian womanhood were both contained in, and explained by, the functional disorder of hysteria. It is interesting, then, that when the twentieth-century feminist critic Catherine Clément explores woman's cultural history through the exemplum and metaphor of the hysteric, she describes a process whereby 'all the history written in feminine mythologies' is repeated in the cycles in which woman is also trapped.[60] Given Caroline's new disappointment at Robert's determination to uproot the copse and turn the green natural spaces of the women's beloved ravine into paved streets macadamized with cinders from the mill, not to mention the ominous presence of the embittered Mrs Pryor in the marital home, Brontë's conclusion bleakly testifies to the inevitability of just such a cycle of repetition.

[58] Tess Cosslett explores the relationship between Caroline and Shirley as central to Brontë's critique of marriage. See *Woman to Woman: Female Friendship in Victorian Fiction* (Brighton: Harvester Press, 1988).

[59] The phrase used by Sandra M. Gilbert to describe the return of the hysteric to 'normality' as defined by men. See Hélène Cixous and Catherine Clément, *The Newly Born Woman*, trans. by Betsy Wing (Manchester: Manchester University Press, 1986. First published as *La Jeune Née*, Paris, 1975), p. xii.

[60] Catherine Clément, *The Newly Born Woman*, p. 4.

FROM PASSION TO PARALYSIS: HYSTERICAL
PATHOLOGY AND DICKENS'S WOMEN

If Dickens's Mrs Clennam has anything in common with
Brontë's Caroline Helstone or MacDonald's Adela Cathcart it is
that all of these fictional invalids turn their disappointed hopes
into somatic disease. But where, with Caroline, we are made
conscious of her transformation of confusion into pain, with
Mrs Clennam we have little sense of an inner experience of
suffering. Instead, like the medical observer, we are left to figure
the state of her mind by interpreting the external signs manifested on the body. And where Caroline struggles for most of
the novel with the mental suffering caused by the cultural
requirement of repression, Mrs Clennam turns repression into
her defining feature, anaesthetizing her body against the painful
demands of social interaction. Mrs Clennam takes prescriptive
femininity to its literal extremes so that the desirable qualities of
quiescence, domesticity, and moral guardianship expected of the
'angel in the house' are travestied in the paralysed body and the
recluse's cell.

When Arthur Clennam returns to the house after his absence
abroad, he finds his mother reclining on a 'black bier-like sofa
. . . propped up behind with one great angular black bolster, like
the block at a state execution' (45). This picture of leisured
languor is a dark parody of middle-class domesticity, a bold and
shocking travesty of 'Home Comforts', the emblematic homecoming scene depicted on the frontispiece of Sarah Stickney
Ellis's *The Women of England*. Arthur's homecoming is marked
by the very absence of 'home comforts' for, upon entering his
mother's room, his senses are assaulted with the 'smell of black
dye in the airless room, which the fire had been drawing out of
the crape and stuff of the widow's dress for fifteen months, and
out of the bier-like sofa for fifteen years'. His mother's touch
was frozen, glassy, and rigid after fifteen years of subduing her
own feelings, not to the superintendence of domestic affairs, but
to the correction of moral weakness. And when she explains to
Arthur how 'The world has narrowed to these dimensions', it is
not mind-numbing domesticity that has reduced the world to a
cell. The implication is rather that, in her commerce with the

outside world through the family business, she has misappropriated the domestic space. Of course, the physical symptoms of which she complains; 'my rheumatic affection, and what with its attendant debility or nervous weakness—names are of no matter now—I have lost the use of my limbs' (46), may well have their origins in sorrow in the same way as other fictional invalids. But where Dickens's representation differs is in that Mrs Clennam, like Miss Havisham in *Great Expectations*, far from trying to conceal her passions, makes a spectacle of them. Even the sofa which, in 'Home Comforts' formed the focal point of maternal loving care, is here compared to the block at a state execution—a very public spectacle of punishment. Mrs Clennam and Miss Havisham externalize their disappointed hopes, making their loss perpetually visible by extending the moment of its origination into a living experience. The wedding dress of the one and the widow's weeds of the other are worn with a vengeance which transmutes them from being mere reflectors of status, and therefore appropriate to women, to unseemly conspicuous displays. Dickens's passionate women are condemned whether they parade their passions or conceal them. Repression, as medical literature has already shown, was as deleterious as expression, and Dickens's fiction is well supplied with women whose emotional repression has, over time, turned into a self-consuming mental malady which mimics consumptive disease.

In complete contrast to the fading beauties of nineteenth-century art and literature, these are the negative images of embittered, resentful women who punish their own bodies into warped and wasted figures of hatred, jealousy, and revenge. Miss Wade, the tormented orphan governess in *Little Dorrit*, whose passion is all the more remarkable, according to the narrator, for being 'so much under her restraint' (632), shows all the signs of a self-consuming sickness. Behind the dead walls, the dead shrubs, and the dry fountain, she lives with Tattycoram in a relationship at once emotionally dependent and mutually destructive—'each proudly cherishing her own anger; each, with a fixed determination, torturing her own breast, and torturing the other's' (634). Miss Wade's self-confessed thoughts of the torturer's rack (636), in their echoes of the state executioner's block, link disappointed women in a psychopathology of passion by which they publicly transgress the boundaries of approved womanhood. Once again, it is the revelation of suffering as opposed to quiet endurance which is the butt of Dickens's disapproval.

At the same time, it could be argued that Mrs Clennam's cloistered invalidism pushes patience and endurance to ridiculous excess. Her paralysed confinement within the inhospitable home subverts the ideals of prescriptive femininity and domestic sanctuary, not so much through defiance and rejection of systems and codes, but by making a spectacle of their inadequacy. Simply to argue, however, that Mrs Clennam's invalidism is a gesture of protest is to run the risk of marginalizing her as an eccentric recluse, and to fail to take account of the extent to which her aberrant wilfulness exposes the formulaic system upon which cultural stereotyping rests. For doctors, the root of the problem of interpreting what they considered to be socially inappropriate behaviour in women lay in the troublesome question of the female will.

It was a cultural given, and one which was later reinforced by evolutionary biologists, that woman, by nature, did not initiate, but reacted. The supposed weakness of the female will was believed to be the reason for this dynamic inequity. But all attempts to define the difference between 'will' meaning volition and 'will' meaning wilfulness collapsed in transparent wordplay or blatant prejudice. Throughout the first half of the century, the notion of woman's weak will, evidenced in her emotional, intuitive, and impulsive nature, existed simultaneously with a suspicion that some women had too strong a will. The spectre of the strong-willed, self-assertive woman offended the preferred image of Victorian womanhood. Doctors writing on hysterical maladies had no difficulty in, on the one hand, ascribing most female functional disorders to the weakness of a woman's will and, in the same article, berating female hysterics with accusations of stubborn resistance to authority and the wilful manufacturing of symptoms. Even the mild-mannered John Conolly had referred, in his disquisition on hysteria, to a wilfulness on the part of some of his female nervous patients which needed to be quelled before they could be restored to health. This timely advice did not go unheeded by less sympathetic doctors who, despite the lack of clinical evidence, stretched the observation to link strong will to moral transgression. With only limited knowledge of psychological cause, many doctors interpreted the phenomenon of hysterical mimesis of organic disease as deliberate and attention-seeking deceit by the hysterical patient. Spasms, convulsions, paralysis, and anaesthesia were all within the repertoire of the determined hysteric. In Dickens's novel, the matter of Mrs Clennam's will is repeatedly addressed but obscured in ambiguity as her observers try to make sense of her impressive resolve and her stubborn seclusion.

Wavering between these contradictory interpretations, the text alerts the reader to the language and images of socially and medically prescribed female roles, but the diagnostic chain linking health to conformity and disease to transgression remains knotted and convoluted. A distinction is undoubtedly implied between the wilful abandonment of a woman's proper participation in social organization and the dedicated fortitude and resolution which Mrs Clennam demonstrates in her execution of her perceived moral duty. But here, obligation that is carried to excess amounts to subversion and is as punishable an offence as refusal. In general terms, the narrator condemns the cloistered life as an aberrant act:

To stop the clock of busy existence, at the hour when we were personally sequestered from it; to suppose mankind stricken motionless, when we were brought to a stand-still; to be unable to measure the changes beyond our view, by any larger standard than the shrunken one of our own uniform and contracted existence; is the infirmity of many invalids, and the mental unhealthiness of almost all recluses.   (331)

Whilst unequivocal in its censure, the passage leaves open the question of agency, and it is a moot point whether 'infirmity' and 'mental unhealthiness' are constitutional weaknesses or the products of stubborn resistance. None the less, it remains true that Mrs Clennam's self-imprisonment transgresses the boundaries of appropriate female behaviour, not so much in cutting herself off from the world of men as in shaping that world to her own terms within the domestic cell, using her sickroom to conduct the business of Clennam and Co.

Mrs Clennam's self-representation of a life not chosen, but

shaped by indoctrination and determined by circumstance, has a powerful validity. Her moral strength is impressive, pushing to excess the role of guardian of the moral conscience both for the family and for the Limited Company of 'Clennam'. As Rigaud Blandois mischievously recalls, it was old Gilbert Clennam who selected her as a suitable wife for his weak and irresolute nephew precisely because of her training in the rigid and unremitting principles imparted through puritanical doctrines of 'wholesome repression, punishment, and fear' (739). In this woman, relates Blandois, Clennam recognized 'a lady of strong force of character, like myself: a resolved lady, a stern lady, a lady who has a will that can break the weak to powder' (737), a lady who was well qualified, it appeared, for a life devoted to the correction of male moral weakness.

But even as she executes her perceived obligation to the moral cleansing of the family as befits her appointment, her persistent demonstration of the toll upon the body of this life-long duty undermines the standard articulations of woman's willingness and fittedness to perform such a role. A life of dedication to the moral and spiritual welfare of others was, for 'Woman', her special privilege and not a hardship, proclaimed the French thinker Auguste Comte. The 'moderating function which is appropriate to Woman', he writes, is her 'happy social position' and 'personal vocation'.[61] Comte's words echoed down the century and across nations, cultures, and disciplines. At first glance, there is a seeming compliance with this notion of privilege in Mrs Clennam's declaration that she deems it 'a grace and favor to be elected to make the satisfaction I am making here' (348). However, her qualification that satisfaction derives not from a sense of service but rather from the certain knowledge that there is no relief from the 'gloom, and hardship, and dark trial', which must be borne with outward stoic impassivity, puts an ironic twist on the idealized concept of a woman's happy and willing self-sacrifice. Crucially, it is her belief that wrongdoing must be everlastingly revenged that gives meaning to her infirmity. Her bodily paralysis is the only guarantee that pain and suffering can be kept in abeyance. 'My affliction', she

[61] Auguste Comte, *The Positive Philosophy*, trans. by Harriet Martineau, 2 vols. (London: Trübner, 1875), ii. p. 113.

explains to Blandois, on his first visit, 'might otherwise have had no meaning to me' (348).

It can equally be argued, of course, that to put such a personally meaningful construction upon her confinement is to underwrite her own delusions, seizing 'the occasion to argue with some invisible opponent' (348) in order to justify her withdrawal from the world. Her words, 'to be elected', are significant inasmuch as they reinforce her conviction that she has no choice but to obey a call from some higher authority. Like the cloistered nun chosen by God, Mrs Clennam regards her own retreat from social life not as willed but as a willingly undertaken response to a requirement to make daily reparation for human folly. Emphatically though, Mrs Clennam is no idealized vision of the household nun and the light in a spiritual and moral darkness. The product of a childhood hardened by the unyielding retributive principles espoused in Old Testament doctrines of the Law of the Father and held in 'The Book', she returns time and again to that authority with ever renewed vehemence. Her account of her early life is a crushing testimony to the regime of 'repression, punishment, and fear' which has made her into the woman described by Blandois as 'without pity, without love, implacable, revengeful, cold as the stone, but raging as the fire' (737).

This image of a woman whose 'implacable', 'cold' exterior masks a 'raging' internal fire recalls Brontë's lesson on enduring the scorpion's sting 'without a sob', and Eagleton's related comments on the contradiction for women between the public mask and the private agony.[62] Like Brontë's, Dickens's model of female suppression of feelings is in tune with contemporary sociomedical dictates which warned of the dangers of inexpressible passion. As J. G. Millingen put it, '[i]n woman, the concentration of her feelings (a concentration that her social position renders indispensable) adds to their intensity; and like a smouldering fire that has at last got vent, her passions, when no longer trammelled by conventional propriety, burst forth in unquenchable violence'.[63] But where Caroline Helstone struggled with her own

---

[62] *Shirley*, p. 128; Terry Eagleton, *Myths of Power*, p. 57.

[63] J. G. Millingen, *Mind and Matter, Illustrated by Considerations on Heredity, Insanity, and the Influence of Temperament in the Development of the Passions* (London: H. Hurst, 1847), pp. 157–8.

sexual awakening in a repressive social regime, Mrs Clennam's body takes upon itself the legacy of others' immoderation. Daily mortification has, in the end, turned to a self-consuming process whereby the exertions of the will have sapped the body's vital energies. An endless ritual of negation which attends the close cell of sexual and sensual sublimation paradoxically focuses attention upon the very physicality of the body it is working to deny. As with Caroline, desire is deadlocked in a cycle of resurgence and repression, and the sexual subject renews itself only to be again subdued.[64] But although the rituals of renewal and correction constitute a crucial factor in the nervous pathology of Mrs Clennam's body, she is no fragile, consumptive invalid. Her illness, unlike Caroline's, is marked with deliberation and willed intention. Flintwinch's remarks upon her resolution, and his regrets that 'if there had been less resistance in her', he might have 'screwed it [her morbid thoughts] out of her' (331), attest to a wilfulness in the duration of her indisposition.

Running counter to the reading of her debility as the sign and consequence of an injunction to oversee the moral management of the family is the possibility that her sickness and seclusion are strategies of resistance in a consciously constructed creative option. Seizing the initiative, she turns the qualities of patience and endurance from requirements of quiescent female virtue into visible demonstrations of the injustice and wrongdoing of men. By this action, she breaks all the rules of female passivity and invisibility. Once again, the links with Miss Havisham are unmistakable. Both women invert the dominant cultural prescription of selfless female devotion to the amelioration of the trials and torments incurred by men in their world of activity and progress, and focus attention instead into their cells of private tragedy. Making a mockery of the idealized vision of the home as a place of spiritual and moral refreshment, they turn themselves into agents of retribution and their homes into

[64] It was Michel Foucault who argued that the notion of the nineteenth century as a one-way dynamic of sexual repression should be abandoned. Instead, he hypothesized, it was a period in which the sexual subject is continually re-affirming itself, paradoxically, through the very mechanisms of self-regulation which social, governmental, and scientific operations on the body as objects of knowledge compelled. *The History of Sexuality*, vol. 1, trans. by Robert Hurley (Harmondsworth: Penguin, 1981. First published 1976), pp. 64–73.

houses of correction. Their atrophied bodies, neither quite dead nor quite alive, parody the figure of the wronged or deserted woman by stubbornly bearing the signs of their injury, thus making their disappointment everlastingly present to themselves and to the gaze of others.[65]

The crucial factor in the onset and prolongation of Mrs Clennam's paralysis is her preoccupation with the past. Paradoxically, in order to keep the overwhelming passions associated with the past under control, she must attend to their subjugation daily. Dickens's depiction of hysterical paralysis that is causally linked to a refusal to let go of the past is no mere literary whim. On the contrary, almost every treatise on hysteria written between the early nineteenth century and the Edwardian period gives serious and detailed consideration to the morbid dwelling on past emotions as a prime cause of intractable psychosomatic disease. It is no coincidence, furthermore, that the novelist, the medical writer, and the social commentator attributed the persistence of the disease to the stubbornness of the patient. Domination by emotions, the injunction on expression, unhealthy fixity in the past, and unfeminine obstinacy were all wheeled together to produce a model of the hysteric as a disruptive force. She upset the established norms of gender hierarchy by selfishly locking herself away from present social integration and from medical help. Almost invariably, medical textbooks warned of cases which turned into a protracted battle of wills ending only when the hysteric was brought back into line by rational, and male, medical authority. Some merely advised inducements or even ridicule to restore 'reason and subordination'.[66] Thomas Laycock took a more radical approach to what he called

---

[65] Similar processes can be seen to work in other texts. In Charlotte Brontë's *Villette*, for instance, Miss Marchmont has turned tragic loss (the death of a fiancé) into a protracted affliction. As the rituals which attend her infirmity daily renew the memory of the pain, her loss is displaced onto her crippled frame. In Anthony Trollope's *Barchester Towers*, the invalid La Signora Madeline Vesey Neroni fashions, from the selfsame construction of inherent debility which harnessed women to their bodies, her own mechanism of power. Requiring to be transported through life on a sofa, she achieves the attention and self-assertion she craves while remaining within a circumscribed role.

[66] F. C. Skey, *Lectures on Hysteria* (London: Longmans, Green, Reader, and Dyer, 1867), pp. 62–3.

'hysterical cunning' by treating, apparently successfully, the 'erotic, self-willed, and quarrelsome' patients in his charge to 'a course of galvanism directed through the ovaria, and by suitable medication and moral and hygienic treatment'.[67] Robert Brudenell Carter's interpretation of the self-willed hysteric is given more detailed consideration over the following pages.

Dickens's censorious remarks with regard to 'the infirmity of many invalids, and the mental unhealthiness of almost all recluses' (331) attribute the intractable cycle of psychosomatic disease to the deliberate renewal of symptoms. The invalid continues to inhabit the moment which first shocked her into seizure by making her body the visible sign and bearer of that moment. Jules Michelet, similarly, directs his eloquent venom at widows who, like Mrs Clennam, turn their memories of past experiences into a strategy of adjournment from an unpalatable present. Holding forth on the state of widowhood, he conjures an insalubrious realm which fits seamlessly into his larger scheme of feminine history wherein womanhood is a pathological condition. The source of their malady, he proclaims, lies in their stubborn, retrogressive, and self-indulgent fixity in the past. Impervious to attempts to coax them back to present reality, they develop an *idée fixe*, a sick obsession by which they adjourn from life, making themselves martyrs to aborted dreams.[68]

Robert Carter is only one of many physicians to make an explicit causal connection between a locked-in preoccupation with the past and patterns of behaviour consistent with hysteria. But, unlike the majority, Carter makes a special point of distinguishing between the recollection of objects or events from the past and the reproduction of the feelings associated with those objects and events. This distinction is an important one

---

[67] Described by Laycock's reviewer in Anon., 'Woman in Her Psychological Relations', p. 34.

[68] *La Femme*, p. 302. Throughout the century, this notion of the *idée fixe* resurfaces time and again. James Cowles Prichard refers to it in a treatise on 'monomania', written for the purposes of clarification in legal trials, in which he argues that possession by one exclusive idea is a mark of the insane. See Chapter 3, n. 82. Ilza Veith points out that Pierre Janet, a disciple of J. M. Charcot, regarded hysteria as invariably characterized by the *idée fixe*, which he described as a stubborn preoccupation with one's own ideas and feelings. See *Hysteria: The History of a Disease*, p. 252.

because it sheds light on the diagnostic borderline where healthy reminiscence turns to morbid reproduction. By far the greater number of sufferers from the morbid condition of revival are women, observes Carter.[69] When, stirred by sentiment or excited by emotions directly emanating from 'objects perceived, or remembered, or imagined', a woman allows her feelings to erupt, it is in that moment of weakness that the thread of healthy life is severed and she is precipitated into a chronically pathological state.[70] From that moment of initial trauma, the frequency with which its associated feelings are regenerated is directly determined by the extent of the patient's intention to prolong her illness. It is at this point, according to Carter, that an unwished-for emotional crisis is turned by the invalid into a self-serving indisposition. When remembered feelings can be reproduced at will, a performative factor in hysterical disorder cannot be ignored, and the stage is set for a drama of confrontation between introspection and disclosure, disguise and exposure, on the parts of patient and practitioner.

As the hysteric grows inured to her pathological fate, her identity is shaped according to the 'parade of illness, and the sympathy consequent upon it'.[71] Most importantly, Carter claims, the drama of hysterical mimesis and the skilful deception of the patient are maintained 'through the instrumentality of the memory, by a direct effort of the will'.[72] In Carter's judgement, such self-indulgent attention-seeking is a form of 'moral delinquency', which, if allowed free rein, transmutes nervous disorder into a consummate art.[73] Juggling these vexed issues of will and culpability, of remembering and display, brings back into focus the fictional representations of Mrs Clennam and Miss Havisham, whose strategies of remembrance have, over time, settled into hollow charades. Of Mrs Clennam, Gillian Beer has noted that it is her 'crazed clinging' to the 'vengeful

[69] It might be noted here that 'nostalgia' was once classified as a category of disease (in William Cullen's famous *Nosology* compiled at the end of the eighteenth century). Although listed under the pining and wasting disorders, nostalgia was diagnosed mostly in men as it was believed to be a disease afflicting the serving soldier who dreamed too much of home. See K. Daly, 'A Study of Nostalgia and Cosmopolitanism in Relation to the Works of Byron', unpublished Ph.D. thesis, (University of Leeds, 1996).

[70] Carter, *On The Pathology and Treatment of Hysteria*, p. 28.

[71] Ibid., pp. 42–3.   [72] Ibid., p. 46.   [73] Ibid., p. 147.

repetitiveness' of memory demanded by the motto 'Do Not Forget' on her husband's watch, which 'stultifies her own life and those of others', and precludes the possibility of growth and change.[74] Both of these Dickensian women divert the acute pain of rejection and loss into the chronic torpor of the body.

The views of the fiction writer and the physician on the pathological consequences of female reminiscence are, in some important respects, neatly mutually confirming. But they are also poised over a contradiction that is rooted in the matter of the dividing line between required and morbid behaviour. Inwardness, devotion, adjournment, and endurance are, for women, it appears, simultaneously the hallmarks of virtue and the potential tools of the hysteric. The paralysed body is, then, the ultimate expression of changelessness and passivity and a gesture of defiance. In the absence of legitimate verbal expression, the body externalizes its passions while conforming to the requirement of silence and suppression. Putting a positive construction on this process of externalization, Catherine Clément celebrates the body of the hysteric as the medium of protest. In the act of remembering her passions and her pain, she transforms her body into 'a theater for forgotten scenes'.[75] Although, for Clément, this facility for release represents woman's spectacular resistance to her relegation to a life of invalidism instituted by the male medical establishment, the performer remains trapped in repetition. Confined by the theatrical space of the body, her language of gestures or of immobility endlessly reconfirms her sickness. Just like Robert Carter's wilful hysteric, the more convincing her performance, the more she condemns herself as sick. And as Carter sees his role as one of masterful intervention in the histrionic cycle, so in Dickens's narrative, Rigaud Blandois assumes a physician's knowing arts to triumph at last over the obstinate grip of a self-generated infirmity.

When, towards the end of *Little Dorrit*, Rigaud Blandois begins to divulge the Clennam 'history of a strange marriage,

---

74 Gillian Beer, 'Origins and Oblivion in Victorian Narrative', in Ruth Bernard Yeazell (ed.), *Sex, Politics and Science in the Nineteenth-Century Novel*, Selected Papers From the English Institute, 1983–4 (Baltimore: Johns Hopkins University Press, 1986), pp. 63–87 (p. 80).

75 *The Newly Born Woman*, p. 5.

and a strange mother, and a revenge, and a suppression' (736), he makes explicit the connection between the suppressed family secrets and Mrs Clennam's paralysed body. Claiming to be 'something of a doctor', Blandois proceeds to take the invalid's pulse and to observe the 'changes' of her malady. The more Blandois reveals about the deceiving husband, his mistress, the child, and the 'scheme of retribution' undertaken by Mrs Clennam, the faster her pulse beats and the more her frozen limbs begin to release themselves. Like the doctor he claims to be, Blandois explains the meaning of her symptoms by drawing upon his privileged knowledge of the aetiological history of her affliction.

Urged on by Blandois, Mrs Clennam breaks out of the prison of paralysis which has confined her for twelve years. No longer able to contain the smouldering passions within her frozen frame, she tells the story which confirms Blandois's diagnosis. Little by little, Mrs Clennam's body yields its pathological secrets to the knowing physician. The mysteries surrounding Arthur's birth, Mrs Clennam's demand that the infant be handed over to her, the cruel, lifelong injunction against the child's real mother, and the withholding of Gilbert Clennam's bequest all emerge from the widow's own lips. As Blandois breaks down her resistance, 'it was noticeable', comments the narrator, that although '[m]any years had come, and gone, since she had had the free use even of her fingers', she 'more than once struck her clenched hand vigorously upon the table, and that when she said these words she raised her whole arm in the air, as though it had been a common action with her' (741). At last, prompted by the wish to spare Arthur from reading the truth of his identity in the papers, letters, and records which, it seems, Flintwinch has kept all along in the house of dark secrets, Mrs Clennam takes flight to the Marshalsea to present her own testimony to Arthur's putative guardian, Amy Dorrit.

Her journey not only propels her violently from stasis to movement, but traverses the uncertain borders between the familiar and the uncanny, dreaming and reality, past and present, and brings into climactic confrontation the gendered and hierarchized modes of existence hitherto kept apart by her protective sickroom walls. A 'spectral' figure is observed making its way through the crowd in the street, drawing all eyes after it, to gaze at its strangeness:

Made giddy by the turbulent irruption of this multitude of staring faces into her cell of years, by the confusing sensation of being in the air and the yet more confusing sensation of being afoot, by the unexpected changes in half-remembered objects, and the want of likeness between the controllable pictures her imagination had often drawn of the life from which she was secluded, and the overwhelming rush of the reality, she held her way as if she were environed by distracting thoughts, rather than by external humanity and observation.   (751)

The configuration of crossings and mergings woven into this passage registers, in the very dissolution of boundaries, the artificiality of binary structural perceptions. Its focal point is the woman as 'spectre', spectacle, and 'other', dislocated from the context of the immediate present. This central image of displacement evokes and communicates other dichotomies, such as disorder and control, normality and deviancy, imagination and concreteness, enclosure and exposure. An opposition of secluded inertia and what is perceived as 'normal', linear progress is suggestive of the gendered duality of existence represented in terms of internality and externality. But Dickens's models elude easy categorization into positively or negatively charged binaries and instead remain fluid.

It is worth recalling for a moment the negative image of the woman as invalid and recluse, sequestered in her dreary abode, turning, as if on a treadmill, whilst outside healthy and normal activity proceeds. Mrs Clennam and Miss Havisham are each represented by Dickens as inhabiting a 'cell' of changelessness, each thinking to 'stop the clock of busy existence' (*Little Dorrit*, 331), to suspend linear history. The gendered model of a cell of changelessness within change is overturned as both women turn the rituals of their entrapment into a histrionic art. Mrs Clennam's stubborn resistance to change is first seen to work as a strategy of selfhood which is both the origin and source of her infirmity. 'The house in the city preserved its heavy dullness', we are told, 'through all [the] transactions' of a business or a personal nature which propel the world outside. Meanwhile, 'the invalid within it turned the same unvarying round of life. Morning, noon, and night, morning, noon, and night, each recurring with its accompanying monotony, always the same reluctant return of the same sequences of machinery, like a dragging piece of clockwork' (331). While the imagery of the 'dragging piece of clockwork' is suggestive of the dreary cycle of the ritual of the female sickroom, it is equally evocative of the world of work and of the repetitive drudgery of factory production. Change in itself is not unreservedly positive, moreover, but tends, inevitably, to collapse and decay:

The wheeled chair had its associated remembrances and reveries, one may suppose, as every place that is made the station of a human being has. Pictures of demolished streets and altered houses, as they formerly were when the occupant of the chair was familiar with them; images of people as they too used to be, with little or no allowance made for the lapse of time since they were seen; of these, there must have been many in the long routine of gloomy days.   (331)

By suppressing all trace of human sensibility to the point of fusion with the wheeled chair, the body has become, as it were, incorporated into the mechanical object. Indistinguishable from the machine, this body retains the power to suspend linear time and preserve the individual's preferred vision of the world. In spite of the critique of the invalid and recluse in the passage as a whole, there is a sense that to retreat into a private world of reminiscence, repetition, and adjournment is itself an insurance against the ineluctable acceleration towards collapse and death. The moment the invalid takes flight from the chair, detaches herself from her own fossilized past, the deadlock is broken and her control over the suspension of history is forfeited.

Where Caroline's return from the temporary suspension of the sickroom, to the 'rude' march of history, is accomplished in resignation, Mrs Clennam's flight from her 'cell of years', from stasis to movement, from past to present, is effected in violent shock and ends in a punishing sentence. Her consciousness is assailed with the terrifying disjunction between her memory and present reality, between the 'controllable pictures' frozen in her imagination, yet endlessly recoverable, and the 'unexpected changes' which time had wrought upon the 'things' themselves in the lapse of time since her withdrawal. In many respects, these intertwinings of the spatial and temporal dimensions in Dickens's writing impugn the simple binaries laid out in medical and cultural-historical definitions of female conformity and transgression. They call into question, even as they underwrite, the precept that the key to psychological stability and physical well-being is to control one's memories and to keep the feelings associated with them quietly suppressed. For the eponymous 'newly born woman' of Cixous and Clément's book, there will be ways out, ways of transcending the mythical, emblematic roles in which she is already inscribed in history. But for Mrs Clennam, newly born from her still-life, there is only a further confinement, a prison of immobility preventing both her return to the past she has just abandoned and her enrolment in the present. Having completed her mission to the Marshalsea, she retraces her steps with Amy only to be engulfed in the débris of the house which finally collapses from its, and her, terminal disease. Blackened and unrecognizable, Mrs Clennam survives but, confined to her wheeled chair for a period of three years, she 'lived and died a statue' (757). If her earlier paralysis was a hysterical imitation of organic disease, a display of Robert Carter's 'willed hysteria', she is punished for her deception by having the real disease 'enforced upon her' (757), so that she lives out the remainder of her days in a mute and catatonic state, detached from the life she had chosen to eschew. Simulating disease in an attempt to draw attention to oneself is, states Carter, 'likely to hasten the arrival of that last epoch in the history of simulative hysteria, when the attention necessary from the malingerer brings its own retribution, and actually produces the morbid condition which she has feigned'.[76] Dickens's 'author'-ization of Mrs Clennam's punishment, and the medical man's authoritative prognosis for the deceiving hysteric, show a remarkable consistency of view.

If Brontë is unable to answer, with any measure of satisfaction, Caroline's questions about her role as a woman, Dickens has fewer reservations. Mrs Clennam's seizure is presented as just punishment for her histrionic pretence of paralysis. But in the broader picture of transgressive femininity, it is a nemesis for her impiety in reversing the 'natural' order of things and usurping the power which is the prerogative of men. In response to her questions as to what else she could have done, the narrator fulminates against her monstrous vanities. When she 'breathed her own breath into a clay image of her Creator', she made of

[76] *On the Pathology and Treatment of Hysteria*, p. 94.

her 'own bad passions', the 'most daring, gross, and shocking images of the Divine nature' (740). Miss Havisham is similarly denounced as a woman who seized upon the masculine construction of a woman's role as guardian of the moral conscience and turned it into the instrument of her own authority. Her immolation in a fireball matches Mrs Clennam's burial alive as a suitably dramatic ending to a performance which has grown wearily anachronistic. It is presented by Dickens as a punishment for a woman who wilfully subverted the ideological framework of appropriate gender spheres. Vengeance notwithstanding, Miss Havisham's error is located in her withdrawal from social obligation: 'that, in shutting out the light of day, she had shut out infinitely more; that, in seclusion, she had secluded herself from a thousand natural and healing influences; that, her mind, brooding solitary, had grown diseased, as all minds do and must and will that reverse the appointed order of their Maker'.[77] These judgements seem clear endorsements of the alleged connection between female social transgression and disease. However, the paradox remains that Dickens's women are sick because they presume to defy an ideological model of womanhood as the uncomplaining guardian angels of the domestic sphere and because they perform their allotted parts within that model with a terrifying conviction.

[77] Charles Dickens, *Great Expectations* (1860–1), ed. by Edgar Rosenberg (New York: W. W. Norton, 1999), p. 297.

CHAPTER TWO

Nervous Sensibility and Ideals of Manliness

THE DISORDER OF LITERARY MEN

An article in *Blackwood's Magazine* in 1869 invites its readers to consider that the 'vapours, fears, and tremors' which seize everyone from time to time hold sway over some individuals to such devastating effect that they seldom find relief from the 'fantastical purgatory' of nervous dreads.[1] The article, attributed to Anne Mozley, continues with the observation that these 'waking fits of morbid depression' are manifestations of a capricious, self-absorbed, and irresolute nature. Purporting to challenge the blanket assumption of women's greater vulnerability to the tyranny of nerves, Mozley argues that only those who are allowed to indulge their 'weaker, more susceptible organisation' are responsible for the stereotype that has come to define the whole of the female sex.[2] Her case, however, is itself undermined by being predicated on the ubiquitous gender stereotypes which typically assigned the characteristics of self-absorption and irresolution to the allegedly weaker organization of women and credited men with the will-power and reason with which to surmount them. But the undeniable incidence of nervous disorder among men as well as women in this so-called 'century of nerves' prompted the formation of new categories of disease which, rather than undermine the much-acclaimed male capacity for self-regulation, sought to separate the collapse of the exhausted man of business from the pitiable imaginings of malingerers and madmen.

[1] 'Vapours, Fears and Tremors', *Blackwood's Magazine*, 105 (1869), 228–37 (p. 228).
[2] Ibid., p. 229.

In the case of women, as we have seen, the inability to subdue the emotions was designated a causal factor in the onset of illness. For men, it was the imagination rather than the emotions which required constant regulation by a controlling will if the stigmatizing symptoms of nervous disease were to be kept at bay. Medically speaking, nervous dreads were the characteristic feature of a condition known as 'hypochondriasis', a disease once believed to constitute a discrete class of diagnosis. For reasons that will become clearer, Victorian doctors began to re-examine the clinical criteria of the disease in the light of contemporary thinking about sexual and social boundaries. Beliefs about essential difference were strengthened by the social, economic, and sexual-political pressures of the period and it was for these, as much as for strictly medical reasons, that doctors were at pains to distinguish hypochondriasis, both causally and symptomatologically, from hysteria. It was generally agreed that the two diseases were definitively male and female maladies. But, despite the efforts of doctors to define and interpret male disease within constructs of masculinity, representations of male nervousness, in medical and literary texts, fashioned an image of an invalid feminized by the very nature of his disease. The perception of the male nervous sufferer was one of a social, sexual, and psychological anomaly in a culture of robust and resolute manliness. Portrayals of hypochondriacal males in fiction work both to highlight and challenge the prevailing definitions of manliness which shaped and fostered this perception. Before proper consideration can be given to these portrayals, however, there are questions that need to be asked about medicine's adaptation of a long-recognized disorder to the new conditions and new sensibilities of Victorian England.

The disease of hypochondriasis can be traced back to humoral pathology and the supposed correspondence between the black bile of melancholy and the visceral organs, principally the gall bladder, liver, and spleen.[3] Nineteenth-century practitioners

---

[3] For a detailed study of the history of nervous and mental diseases from their origins in melancholia and the theory of humours, see Roy Porter, *Mind-Forg'd Manacles: A History of Madness in England from the Restoration to the Regency* (Cambridge, Mass.: Harvard University Press, 1987), pp. 45–9.

argued over the diagnosis of a disorder whose signs and symptoms were to be found across a range from mild indigestion to severe mental alienation verging on insanity. Writing in *The Cyclopaedia of Practical Medicine* in 1833, James Cowles Prichard stresses the complexity of a malady characterized by abdominal discomfort, 'a remarkable lowness of spirits or a desponding habit of mind', an obsession with 'every minute change in the bodily feelings', and apprehension of 'extreme danger from the most trifling ailments'.[4] Although the disease was understood to be a conformation of neurotic and organic elements, Prichard is at pains to establish that, whatever the seat of origin, hypochondriasis is a 'real' disease and not merely a self-indulgent affectation.[5]

Over twenty years later, James Copland's comprehensive study in *A Dictionary of Practical Medicine* scarcely advances medical knowledge though it re-confirms that the symptoms characterizing the disease 'are by no means imaginary':

They evidently depend upon physical disease, in connection with a morbidly exalted state of sensibility. This physical disease commences in the digestive organs, attended with morbid organic sensibility, which extends to the cerebro-spinal nervous system, thereby aggravating and multiplying the morbid phenomena.[6]

Of course, Copland, like others earlier in the century, was drawing on an extensive literature going back to Robert Burton's *Anatomy of Melancholy* (1621) and beyond that to classical times. It had long been accepted that mental and somatic criteria waged a battle of mutual aggravation in their victims but, in

---

[4] J. C. Prichard, 'Hypochondriasis', in J. Forbes, A. Tweedie, and J. Conolly, (eds.), *The Cyclopaedia of Practical Medicine*, 4 vols. (London: Sherwood, Gilbert, Piper *et al*, 1833–5), ii. pp. 548–7 (p. 548).

[5] The title of a treatise by Nicholas Robinson in 1729 suggests that 'hypochondriack melancholy' was understood as a disorder of the physiological nervous system in the eighteenth century: *A new system of the spleen, vapours, and hypochondriack melancholy; wherein all the decays of the nerves, and lownesses of the spirits, are mechanically accounted for. To which is subjoined, a discourse upon the nature, cause and cure of melancholy, madness, and lunacy etc.* (London: 1729, my emphases).

[6] James Copland, *A Dictionary of Practical Medicine: comprising general pathology, the nature and treatment of diseases, morbid structures, and the disorders especially incidental to the climates, to the sex, and to the different epochs of life &c.*, 3 vols. (London: Longman, Brown, Green, Longmans, and Roberts, 1858), ii. pp. 260–1.

identifying predisposing causes, Copland painted a picture of a disease which not only struck the weak, fearful, and introspective, but which lay in wait for the moment when even the exponents of the manly virtues of resolution and perseverance might be overtaken by self-doubt. Among the educated classes, 'mental exertion and fatigue, or prolonged or overstrained attention and devotion to a particular subject', are likely to occasion the disease. It is for this reason that it has often been called 'the disorder of literary men; but whoever is engaged in active mental pursuits, or in departments of business requiring great intellectual exertion, or occasioning anxiety of mind, is equally liable to it'.[7] Despite repeated assertions that hypochondriasis affects 'somewhat oftener the nervous, the melancholic, the sanguine, and the bilious', these words must have brought cold comfort when read in the context of the wide-reaching categories of susceptibility and liability.[8] The point I want to emphasize is the all-encompassing vagueness of a term which, like hysteria, could be invoked to fill the gaps in knowledge along the organic—neurotic—psychological spectrum, and expediently serve a broader agenda wherever ideas of masculinity were reshaping the patterns of disease. After it had been generally accepted that both hysteria and hypochondriasis were functional nervous disorders and not organic diseases, their allocation to one sex or another could no longer be supported. Gradually, hypochondriasis ceased to carry its associations with the abdominal pathology of bilious men, although some of its elements were retained as it was accommodated into the more general, and non-sex-specific, state of anxiety about the body's

---

[7] From the time that Thomas Trotter placed 'literary men' at the top of his list of categories of individuals most likely to suffer from 'dyspepsia, hypochondriasis and melancholia', the term 'the disorder of literary men' is frequently reproduced in medical and social documents throughout the first half of the nineteenth century. See *A View of the Nervous Temperament; being a Practical Enquiry into the Increasing Prevalence, Prevention, and Treatment of Those Diseases Commonly Called Nervous* (London: Longman, Hurst, Rees, Orme, and Brown, 1807), pp. 37–9.

[8] Working-class people could not be assured of immunity. Citing Prichard, Copland notes 'that agricultural labourers, who spend a great portion of their time in solitary employment in the country, are frequently the subjects of this complaint'. Prichard had listed tailors and shoemakers among potential sufferers because the poor posture they are obliged to adopt for their work is likely to occasion 'a torpid state of the intestinal canal'. *The Cyclopaedia of Practical Medicine*, ii. p. 552.

health familiarly known as 'hypochondria'. When William Crimsworth, in Charlotte Brontë's *The Professor*, suffers an attack of 'Hypochondria', he is suddenly gripped by a malady, the acuteness of which is puzzling to a modern reader. The one element in Brontë's depiction of the disease which strikes a common chord both with medical definitions of hypochondriasis and the popular understanding of hypochondria is that Crimsworth's dread of being mentally and physically overtaken by some indefinable but irresistible force is more debilitating than any palpable symptoms. Implicit in Brontë's representation of the incidence of hypochondria is its association with morbid introspection and the nervous temperament. But the language and imagery employed to communicate its effects are powerfully indicative of a perception of a disease whose moral, social, and gender implications far exceeded its clinical boundaries. Not that doctors were altogether clear about those boundaries; the precise nature of the complex relationship between organic disease, nervous susceptibility, temperament, and type continued to be a vexed question of medical disputation throughout the century.

Bound up with this question is a more general one about the gendering of illnesses whose origins could no longer, with any degree of scientific integrity, be assigned to biological sex. Disease representation, it has already been noted, is determined as much by current attitudes, prejudices, and assumptions as by the specifics of medical knowledge. Functional disorders, by virtue of their obscure and inexact origins, were particularly subject to modification and, in the absence of structural lesions, their manifold symptoms were continually being reassigned to defects of mental or emotional organization. Literary representations of sufferers of nervous debility work within and against the shifting parameters of disease designation and, in fiction and medicine, the configuration of the male nervous invalid was shaped and informed by the changing perceptions of manliness. Stereotypes of masculinity were no less powerful and pervasive than their feminine equivalents and, like them, worked by reducing variety and complexity to over-simplified standards of appropriate and inappropriate behaviour. In both cases, the terms of gender representation were unstable and the prescriptions for health and respectability were confused and contradictory. As medical men struggled to identify new categories for male maladies which bore alarming resemblances to hysteria, novelists made use of the lack of stable aetiologies to frame narratives of invalidism which imaginatively reinterpret what medical discourse sought to fix and enclose. By exploring the contradictions and ambiguities within medicalized definitions of gender, representations of invalidism in literary texts challenge the defining categories of disease classification. This is true of Charlotte Brontë's *The Professor* and George Eliot's 'The Lifted Veil'. In the novels of Dickens, for example, or the sensation novels of the 1860s, representations of male disorders work not so much through exploration and interrogation as by exaggeration and elaboration of the absurdities arising out of gender stereotypes of disease.

Despite advances in the science of neurology, ideological assumptions preceded diagnosis in case after case of male sickness. The difficulties doctors faced in dealing with nervously ill men were due in large part to the seeming inseparability of formulations of disease and measurements of manliness. Importantly, too, these writings give clear indication of the way in which distinctions of gender, or more precisely, ideas of what constituted appropriate masculine or feminine characteristics and behaviour, were becoming increasingly the province of medical science. During the period, the medical profession assumed an unprecedented authority for defining the standard and for predicting the dire consequences of falling outside it. Professional textbooks as well as domestic handbooks pointed to a causal connection between deviation from the prescriptions of self-regulation and a whole range of diseases, from nervous dreads to insanity. Eager to promote the virtues of a more vigorous and outgoing ideal of manliness which would meet the demands of a growing industrial economy and an expanding empire, eminent physicians routinely fell back upon long-established gender divisions of reason and feeling, resolution and emotional weakness, culture and nature, when defining the parameters of nervous disease. In a climate which set a premium on bodily vigour, mental toughness, and emotional restraint, it became common practice for alienists and the growing numbers of nerve specialists to validate a clinical distinction between a breakdown of nerve force, with its suitably masculine mechanistic image, and the feminizing neuroses associated with the constitutional hypochondriac.

This distinction was one which was rarely, if ever, made in the early part of the century. While the existence of various forms of neuroses in male subjects is never denied, the disease of hysteria in men is either dismissed on the grounds of its rarity or reclassified according to external, rather than constitutional or temperamental, causes. John Conolly, somewhat ambiguously, notes the extreme improbability of hysteria in males while pointing to the fact that 'few observant practitioners' had not come across it.[9] Of course, Conolly knew that the traditional uterine origins of hysteria no longer made medical sense. But, if this were so, did men suffer the same symptoms, and could their condition properly be called hysterical? It is significant that the cases Conolly goes on to cite, in one way or another, avoid any suggestion of unmanly weakness and susceptibility.

Reasons are assiduously sought whereby these unfortunate victims may be exonerated from the blame which increasingly attaches to male nervous invalids during the course of the century. One case was excused on the grounds that it concerned a 'gentleman' destined for holy orders who, against his natural inclinations, was forced to adopt a life of strict celibacy. Another, that of a boy whose symptoms followed in the wake of a severe fever, is attributed to febrile delirium.[10] Conolly's reference to the observations of a ship's surgeon, a Mr Watson, brings into focus the phenomenon of hysteria in serving soldiers which, as Elaine Showalter has shown, undermined further the gendered categories of nervous afflictions.[11] Conolly quotes

[9] Ibid., ii. p. 567.   [10] Ibid., ii. p. 565.

[11] Showalter notes that, in the First World War, soldiers returning from the front line of battle were exhibiting the symptoms of hysteria, but to name them as such would destabilize the 'ideology of absolute and natural difference between women and men'. Despite the attempts by Charles S. Myers, a laboratory psychologist from Cambridge University, to identify an organic cause for the mental impairment experienced by these men, none could be established, and the term 'shell-shock' was coined to confer a more manly designation upon symptoms markedly consistent with female hysteria. Though the term 'shell-shock' was later dismissed by the medical profession as inadequate, its persistence in popular usage testified to the perceived need for a gender distinction in hysterical disorder. The phenomenon of tens of thousands of 'emotionally incapacitated men' seriously undermined the categories of hysteria, and forced, Showalter remarks, 'a reconsideration of all the basic

Watson, who had, in turn, cited extracts from the following passage in Thomas Trotter's *Medicina Nautica* of 1804:

In my general visit to the fleet at this time, [August 1797] there appeared an unusual despondency and dejection of spirits among the patients. . . . When some of these cases were moved to the hospital-ship, we found not a few of them subject to very frequent fits of hysteria; and where this singular affection recurred with as much violence of convulsion as we have ever marked it in female habits, attended with globus, dysphagia, immoderate risibility, weeping, and delirium. The same sympathy seemed to extend from one to another, as is often met with in the fair sex. . . . I could not explain this extraordinary complaint among our patients in any other way, than resolving it to the effects the late tumults in the fleet had made on the feelings of the people . . . and which had kept them in a state of constant dread and apprehension.[12]

The correspondence of symptoms manifested by traumatized fighting men and hysterical women is not addressed by Conolly as an issue significant in itself, but merely serves to 'set . . . at rest' the question of the existence of male hysteria only in exceptional circumstances.[13]

Some years later, Thomas Laycock's 1840 treatise, *On the Nervous Diseases of Women,* is already less sympathetic towards male sufferers of what is still regarded as essentially a female disease. Commenting on the mere handful of cases that have come to his attention, he makes the point that 'two were fat, pale-faced, effeminate-looking men' whilst another was 'pale and delicate'. Laycock was convinced that it was lack of the power of self-control to curb the 'vicious habits' which excited the brain and debilitated the nervous system that turned men into hysterics by 'reducing the blood to a state similar to

concepts of English psychiatric practice'. *The Female Malady: Women, Madness, and English Culture, 1830–1980* (London: Virago, 1987), pp. 167–9.

[12] Watson, himself a ship's surgeon in the East India Company, refers for precedent to passages from these observations which were made by Trotter during his tenure as Physician to the Fleet of Great Britain in the Napoleonic Wars and recorded in *Medicina Nautica: An Essay on the Diseases of Seamen,* 3 vols. (London: Longman, Hurst, Rees, and Orme, 1804), ii. pp. 28–9. See also 'Mr Watson's Case of Hysteria', *Edinburgh Medical and Surgical Journal,* 11 (1815), 303–4.

[13] *The Cyclopaedia of Practical Medicine,* ii. p. 567.

that of the hysterical female'.[14] Those cases which could not be accounted for either organically or by a lifestyle deemed unnatural by normative standards were more problematic. Writers were divided into those who regarded conditions which 'resembled' hysteria as confined to males with weak, feminine natures, and those who preferred to construe them as manifestations of a different disease altogether. But in spite of the rapid developments in neurological science, the taint of effeminacy which attached to all forms of male nervous disorder was extraordinarily difficult to eradicate. Invariably, medical articles on the subject of nervously ill men used language identical to that of the female stereotype of weak-willed passivity to describe their symptoms. Fiction writers, too, draw on the same association of ideas when they emphasize the feminizing effects upon male characters of a hypersensitive disposition.

It was hardly surprising that ambiguities and contradictions in the gender designation of disease forced evermore elaborate explanations. Frederick Skey, like Conolly, dismisses a direct connection between hysteria and female biology but then, in a significant move, draws men into the frame of 'female malady' by re-siting the causal criteria of male hysteria in a constitutional predisposition and enfeeblement of the will. 'It is notoriously far more common in women than in men', he writes, but does not affect 'persons of either sex who are characterised by vigour of mind, of strong will, of strength and firmness of character'.[15] Robert Brudenell Carter takes the view that, while neither sex is totally exempt, there are very good reasons for supposing that modern civilization and refinement have brought men under the sway of hysteria, rather than that the disease was inaccurately named. It is very likely, he suggests, that 'in rude and barbarous times' the name was appropriately ascribed to a disease peculiar to women, but as the 'circle of masculine emotions' has widened, 'the physical organism has been more and more subjugated to their influence'.[16] Even where there exists at a subtextual level an understanding of its non-sex-specificity, in both medical and

[14] Thomas Laycock, *A Treatise on the Nervous Diseases of Women* (London: Longman, Orme, Brown, Green, and Longmans, 1840), pp. 82–3.
[15] F. C. Skey, *Lectures on Hysteria*, pp. 41–2, 61.
[16] Robert Brudenell Carter, *On the Pathology and Treatment of Hysteria*, pp. 32–3.

literary discourse the phenomenon of hysteria is mediated in one way or another when its subject is male.

In the last decade of the century, the demarcation line between legitimate and illegitimate disease in men becomes much more uncompromisingly drawn as new external conditions prompt the need for a category of nervous breakdown which is quite separate from the morbid affections characteristic of hypochondriasis. An article by Horatio Bryan Donkin on the clinical distinctions between male hysteria and hypochondriasis, intended as a guide for puzzled medical practitioners, leaves its readers with an interpretative dilemma whose happy resolution depends less upon identifying symptoms than upon correctly appraising the sufferer. By linking the range of abnormal sensory and behavioural symptoms to traumatizing experiences encountered in the stressful world of the workplace, male hysteria is made, if not altogether respectable, at least explicable. Thus, '[h]ysteria in men', Donkin observes, 'is frequently a sequela of sudden nervous shocks, such as accidents, explosions, and is often connected with alcoholism. Marked instances of hysteria, . . . have been frequently observed and recorded as occurring after railway accidents'.[17] Cases lacking such obvious traumatic origins are then relegated to a lower order of neurosis which has close associations with female hysteria. But, despite similarities in observable symptoms, hypochondriasis is, according to Donkin, aetiologically distinct from even the milder forms of hysteria. The self-generating and self-perpetuating aspects of hypochondriasis make it even less excusable and the disease, Donkin asserts, is 'marked off from hysteria by its different psychopathy, and is altogether a neurosis of less ample range. The prevailing mental state is that of depression, and the morbid sensations are not, as a rule, excited by any obvious external cause, as is most often the case in hysteria'.[18] From mid-century onward, then, it was those individuals whose symptoms appeared without evident or understandable cause who were most at the mercy of the shifting contours of functional nervous disease.

[17] H. B. Donkin, 'Hysteria', in D. H. Tuke (ed.), *A Dictionary of Psychological Medicine*, 2 vols. (London: John Churchill, 1892), i. p. 624.
[18] Ibid., i. p. 625.

One of the ways in which definitions were adjusted to accommodate nervous disorders in men, whilst at the same time registering an immunity for the vast majority, was by delineating a hysteric constitution. When male sufferers are located in the same referential frame of nervous hypersensitivity, obsessive introspection, and susceptibility to emotional disturbance as their ailing female counterparts, temperament becomes more significant than gender in the diagnostic criteria of hysteria. Jan Goldstein has shown how writers in nineteenth-century France turned the heightened sensitivity and self-absorption associated with the neurotic temperament to their own advantage and, in so doing, revealed the extraordinary adaptability of the interface between medical and literary discourses of gender. Novelists such as Balzac, Stendhal, Flaubert, and Zola found, in the proliferating medical treatises on the psychiatric aetiology of hysteria, a discourse of nervous disorder which could be appropriated to serve the interests of literary sensibility by validating the 'literary' practices of introspection and insight. Flaubert's self-diagnosis of the female disorder of hysteria is one example. A passage from his letter to George Sand in 1867 announces a shift in the perception of hysteria from its specific gender association to a condition of non-gendered hypersensitivity: 'I experience flutterings of the heart for no reason at all—an understandable thing, moreover, in an old hysteric like me. For I maintain that men can be hysterics just like women, and that I am one . . . I have recognized all my symptoms: the ball [rising in the throat], the [sensation of the] nail in the back of the skull'.[19] By partaking of the symptoms of nervous hypersensitivity and vulnerability more usually assumed to be the plight of the hysterical woman, Flaubert succeeds in blurring the boundaries of gender affiliation in order to affirm the androgynous ideal to which he was artistically and intellectually committed. His strategy, as Goldstein argues, is to adapt the phenomenon of hysteria into a discourse of the male, sensitive, creative artist by conceptualizing an analogy between the two. But even if this effectively desexualizes the condition, the very

---

[19] Cited in Jan Goldstein, 'The Uses of Male Hysteria: Medical and Literary Discourse in Nineteenth-Century France', *Representations*, 34 (1991), 134–65 (p. 134).

concept of an analogy between female hysteria and male hyper-sensitivity retains the established gendered categories even as the clinical boundaries shift.[20]

If French psychiatry enabled at least a conceptual destabilization of the gender definitions built into pathology, writers in England were less willing to admit controversial claims into a discourse which, I would argue, had a greater investment in difference. Firstly, there were the narrowly prescriptive attitudes to manliness engendered by a deeply conservative culture. Secondly, the British medical preference for a physiological basis to neurotic disease worked to preserve rather than unsettle the stereotypes.[21] As one medical publication succeeds another, lines are continually being re-drawn in an effort to separate closely similar symptoms into gendered categories of disease designation. Whether male nervous afflictions are inscribed within the available contexts of female hysteria, or framed anew around morbid pathologies held to be specifically male, the attributes of nervousness, acute sensitivity, and enfeebled will epitomized in hysteria ensured the preservation of an ideal of English manliness by banishing men who fell short of that ideal to the realms of effeminate inadequacy.

Novelistic representations of male nervous disorder are predicated upon an assumption and an ideal. Firstly, the conjunction of femininity and sickness, as explored in the previous chapter, made available the stereotype of the hysteric and the notion of a 'female malady'. Men who suffer from nervous disorders with no real or obvious cause are assumed to be reduced to the state

---

[20] Goldstein points out that, despite Flaubert's avid reading of medical resources on hysteria, his frequent references in correspondence, and his self-diagnosis, the word never appears in his novels, which are yet 'suffused with hysteria' (p. 138). It might also be noted that the British physician and alienist John Conolly describes the sensation of the nail to which Flaubert refers, not in the back of the skull but 'that of a nail driven into the forehead', a sensation known as 'clavus hystericus'. See *The Cyclopaedia of Practical Medicine*, ii. p. 561.

[21] The status of male hysteria was a source of controversy in the medical writings of both countries. But it seems that the incidence of the disease in men was more positively acknowledged in France. Later in the century, H. B. Donkin regretted what he considered to be British doctors' neglect of the subject. He writes: 'Recently, the Paris neurologists, and notably M. Guinon, have insisted anew and with characteristic clearness on the frequent existence of hysteria in men, which has been certainly passed over too lightly by many English writers'. See Donkin, 'Hysteria', in *A Dictionary of Psychological Medicine*, i. p. 624.

of women. In Brontë's *The Professor* and Eliot's 'The Lifted Veil', the 'feminine' qualities possessed by the respective heroes are construed as handicaps which disadvantage them in the man's world. Secondly, but not unrelatedly, their predicament lies in their physical and emotional incompatibility with a prevailing ideal of middle-class manliness which is, in turn, bound up with ideas of family and nation. Principles of production, property, and prosperity, espoused by the new manufacturing class on familial and national levels, were powerful contributors to an emerging ideology which marginalized both the 'effeminate' artist and the 'effete' aristocrat on the grounds of their non-contribution to a national, domestic, or sexual economy. Images of a fading gentry community abound, especially in popular fiction, as the social and economic climate banished those whom Jenny Bourne Taylor has called 'the sons of redundant ancient families' to the realms of historical anachronism and physiological degeneration.[22]

Brontë's and Eliot's depictions of male sufferers explicitly and implicitly interrogate the very principles and tenets around which they are framed. Representations of nervously ill men in sensation fiction, a form almost by definition designed to provoke particular responses in the reader, make more calculated use of the prejudices and assumptions which attach to persistent stereotypes. Frederick Fairlie, for instance, in Wilkie Collins's *The Woman in White*, is the creation of a novelist who knew well how to exploit the taint of moral weakness that clung to the nervously sensitive man. As a man of considerable wealth who has no need of gainful employment, Frederick Fairlie could scarcely attribute his delicate constitution to the strains of progress, to the relentless struggle for position which beset the middle-class professional or man of business. Instead, his was the inexcusable kind of affliction which was considered to be self-induced and self-perpetuating. The kind of indisposition in which Fairlie indulges harks back to an age of languid elegance. That drawing-room sensibility, once the mark of civilized refinement, had become an anachronism in an industrial economy where a more muscular manliness was required to meet the

---

[22] Jenny Bourne Taylor, *In the Secret Theatre of Home: Wilkie Collins, Sensation Narrative, and Nineteenth-Century Psychology* (London: Routledge, 1988), p. 70.

demands of the family, the nation, and beyond that, the empire. 'Hypochondriacal bachelors', to borrow Taylor's label, were portrayed as unnatural, unmanly, and un-English.

Living in almost anchorite seclusion in his private sitting room, Fairlie has placed himself out of reach of the productive, reproductive, familial, and economic demands which beleaguer many a mid-century male. The condition from which he purports to suffer is sufficiently non-specific to be dismissed by others as mere selfish affectation, and it is with wry amusement that Marian Halcombe explains to Hartright:

Mr Fairlie is too great an invalid to be a companion for anybody. I don't know what is the matter with him, and the doctors don't know what is the matter with him, and he doesn't know himself what is the matter with him. We all say it's on the nerves, and we none of us know what we mean when we say it.[23]

It is not long before Hartright, too, recognizes 'that Mr Fairlie's selfish affectation and Mr Fairlie's wretched nerves meant one and the same thing' (41). Unlike the eponymous Basil, another of Collins's hypersensitive bachelors, Fairlie displays little of the frantic excitability that exposure to the unfamiliar strains of modern life induces. On the contrary, Hartright's impression of Fairlie's tranquil seclusion is of a 'deliciously soft, mysterious' sensuality in which the man himself, pallid and listless, finds asylum (39).

In the forthright, middle-class man of the time, bent on self-improvement, this fragile specimen of manhood, 'languidly-fretful', with feet 'effeminately small', and clad in 'little woman-ish bronze-leather slippers' arouses a repugnance akin to that felt by medical men for the pitiful figures whose debility they attributed to moral weakness or lack of will. A curiously epicene quality about Fairlie eludes, even as it invites, pathological investigation. There was in his demeanour 'something singularly and unpleasantly delicate in its association with a man, and, at the same time, something which could by no possibility have looked natural and appropriate if it had been transferred to the personal appearance of a woman' (39–40).

---

[23] Wilkie Collins, *The Woman in White* (1860), ed. by John Sutherland (Oxford: Oxford University Press, 1996), p. 34. Subsequent references to this edition will be given in the text.

Although we are meant to read Fairlie's misanthropic view of
the world and his withdrawal from it as characteristic
hypochondriacal symptoms, an authorial critique of that
world's philistinism is only thinly disguised in the representation
of the aesthete to whom the slightest movement or noise has
become 'indescribable torture', and to whom the handling of
money has become exclusively the pastime of the coin collector.
Collins's purposively exaggerated portrait of self-conscious
nervous hypersensitivity in a man who describes himself as
'nothing but a bundle of nerves dressed up to look like a man'
(356) both registers and responds to the broader debate about
the place of celibacy in a culture which, publicly at least, set
such store on matrimony. In his Narrative, Fairlie's annoyance
at having to contribute in the first place stems from his sense of
the injustice of the cruel treatment which single people receive
at the hands of their married contemporaries. Far from being
grateful for the 'considerate and self-denying' choice not to 'add
a family of your own to an already overcrowded population', he
complains, 'you are vindictively marked out by your married
friends, who have no similar consideration and no similar self-
denial, as the recipient of half their conjugal troubles, and the
born friend of all their children' (352). Of course, this is comic.
But behind the comedy lies a familiarity with a concept of
manliness in which those who failed, or chose not, to live in
accordance with its precepts were held in breach of their social
responsibility. Fairlie's account had sobering parallels in real-life
correspondence and memoirs.

Private responses to the way in which bodily vigour and
mental toughness became the hallmarks of manliness reveal the
extent of the psychic and somatic cost to individual males of a
cult of masculinity which appeared to have transformed once
admired qualities of intellectual dedication and sensitivity to the
needs and feelings of others into undesirable weaknesses. In her
discussion of 'Manly Nerves', Janet Oppenheim records a
number of autobiographical accounts of nineteenth-century
sufferers from the 'taint' of effeminacy, a social stigma which
many men found painful and destructive. Among them A. C.
Benson, who, through the character of Hugh in *Beside Still
Waters*, expressed a deep sadness that the time had come when
'the cultivation of art, once deemed perfectly compatible with

manliness, and even heroism, had become "rather a dilettante business", which no self-respecting man would pursue', and when ' "a man occupied in quiet and intellectual pursuits, would be held to be a failure" ' when measured against the more visible and extrovert pursuits of the man of business.[24] Earlier, an anonymous memoir to Samuel Greg, who had suffered a devastating nervous collapse when economic depression shattered all his philanthropic and paternalistic dreams for his factory and workforce, makes the point when it pays tribute to his endearing feminine qualities of compassion and nurturing, whilst simultaneously identifying them as the source of his inadequacy as a man.[25]

Similarly, remarks made in Henry Maudsley's 1866 memoir of his late father-in-law, John Conolly, testify to the rapidity with which the association between sensitivity and unmanliness had taken hold in medical and popular perception. Maudsley's description of Conolly as a man of 'fine sensibilities' begins to seem less than complimentary when offered as the reason for his wavering and shrinking from 'the disagreeable occasions of life'. 'In some respects', writes Maudsley, 'I think, his mind seemed to be of a feminine type; capable of a momentary lively sympathy, which might even express itself in tears' rather than meet difficulties with 'deliberate foresight and settled resolution'. Unfortunately, he continues, character deemed 'most graceful and beautiful in a woman is no gift of fortune to a man having to meet the adverse circumstances and pressing occasions of tumultuous life'.[26] Tenderness and sympathy are incompatible, it seems, with the toughness and combative instincts necessary in a man's world.[27]

In his late novel, *Heart and Science* (1883), Wilkie Collins demonstrates the enduring currency of these ideas when his hero Ovid Vere, himself a physician, begins to suffer from a

[24] Janet Oppenheim, *'Shattered Nerves': Doctors, Patients, and Depression in Victorian England* (New York: Oxford University Press, 1991), p. 179.

[25] Ibid., pp. 179–80.

[26] Henry Maudsley, 'Memoir of the Late John Conolly, M.D.', *Journal of Mental Science*, 12 (1866), 151–74 (pp. 161, 173).

[27] For an interesting reassessment of the concept of separate gender spheres based, more unusually, on the experiences of husbands and fathers, see John Tosh, *A Man's Place: Masculinity and the Middle-Class Home in Victorian England* (New Haven and London: Yale University Press, 1999).

'morbid sensitiveness' which is taken to be the unmistakable sign of the onset of nervous disease. That his sensitivity constituted a threat to his masculinity is made quite explicit when the narrator remarks on how Vere's 'shattered nerves unmanned him, at the moment of all others when it was his interest to be bold. The fear that he might have allowed himself to speak too freely—a weakness which would never have misled him in his days of health and strength—kept his eyes on the ground'.[28] With his reserves of strength already depleted as a result of his recent lack of care for his physical well-being, and the emotional strain of wanting to confess his love for Carmina, the exhausted Vere sinks into a nervous collapse, exacerbated, according to the vivisectionist Dr Benjulia, by weakness of the heart. Of course, it is Collins's concern to show the sensitive and nervously susceptible Ovid Vere, in the end, as the more humane doctor and the better man. But the plot relies for much of its tension on the tacit medical and popular knowledge that emotional sensibility reduces grown men to the feebler condition of women. It is for the very reason of alarm at being continually over-whelmed by emotion beyond his capacity to control it that Vere is obliged to leave for the reviving air of Canada. Reinvigorated 'on the broad prairies and in the roving life', he is able to conquer his tendency to tears and eventually returns from Canada a more masterful man. The 'once tremulous nerves' that undermined his manhood are held at bay by the 'robust vitality that rioted in his blood' and it is with a new resolution that he takes up his manly (as husband to Carmina) and moral (as antivivisectionist doctor) duties with 'dry eyes', no longer moved to womanish tears by birdsong, music, or the shadows of evening on the fields.[29] Collins uses the character of Vere to establish a more humane middle ground between the extremes of 'heart' and 'science', feeling and reason, and, most importantly, to validate the pursuit of medical understanding and better therapeutics through bedside practice rather than through vivisection. Implicit,

---

[28] Wilkie Collins, *Heart and Science: A Story of the Present Time* (1883), ed. by Steve Farmer (Peterborough, Ontario: Broadview Press, 1996), p. 108.
[29] Ibid., p. 304.

however, in the happy resolution of this tale of love and medical science is an understanding that control over the emotions is a precondition of healthy masculinity.

If doctors failed to acknowledge that stereotyped prescriptions of manliness were, of themselves, insidious contributors to male medical problems, it was precisely because the masculine power of will, self-regulation, and control was taken for granted. Men were constantly being reminded that will-power was the property which gave them a natural advantage over women and beasts, and that the prevention of nervous disease was a matter of exerting their superior will. The strength of a man's resolve was the key factor in escaping the kind of vicious circle of infirmity and irresolution of which physicians like John Reid had warned: 'In the class of what are called nervous affections', Reid pointed out, 'it unfortunately happens that the very essence of the disease often consists in a debility of the resolution, that the ailment of body arises from an impotency of the power of resistance.'[30] With every confidence in men's natural ability, the Reverend John Barlow published his Royal Institution papers in a book entitled *On Man's Power Over Himself to Prevent or Control Insanity*, in which he proposed measures for avoiding 'Morbid affections of the nervous system and brain' by applying 'the immense power of the Intellectual force' to prevention and control.[31] Inevitably, such blanket assumptions generated anxiety and guilt among many who felt themselves to be unduly susceptible to depression, so that mutually exacerbating morbid afflictions of body and mind only hastened the slide towards nervous collapse. In her novel *Agnes Grey*, Anne Brontë paints a portrait of a sufferer from precisely this form of psychosomatic reciprocal aggravation.

Through the narratorial voice of Agnes, we learn how her father's guilt about the straitened circumstances into which his imprudent investments have plunged his wife and family intensifies the calamity of his financial losses and exacerbates his symptoms. Despite her mother's uncomplaining support,

---

[30] John Reid, *Essays on Hypochondriasis*, 2nd edn. (London: Longman, Hurst, Rees, Orme, and Brown, 1821), p. 20.

[31] John Barlow, *On Man's Power Over Himself to Prevent or Control Insanity* (London: William Pickering, 1843).

Agnes's father 'was completely overwhelmed'; his 'health, strength, and spirits sank beneath the blow; and he never wholly recovered them'. Remorse was his greatest torment. As 'gall and wormwood to his soul', it undermined his resistance and hastened his decline:

The very willingness with which [his wife] performed these duties, the cheerfulness with which she bore her reverses, and the kindness which withheld her from imputing the smallest blame to him, were all perverted by this ingenious self-tormentor into further aggravations of his sufferings. And thus the mind preyed upon the body, and disordered the system of the nerves, and they in turn increased the troubles of the mind, till by action, and reaction, his health was seriously impaired; and not one of us could convince him that the aspect of our affairs was not half so gloomy, so utterly hopeless as his morbid imagination represented it to be.[32]

In this passage, male nervous disorder is represented, characteristically, as a function of a morbid imagination. As will be seen, imagination was not a faculty to be encouraged in men since it implied a creativity which transgressed the boundaries defining masculine rational control. Here, as elsewhere, the subtext of gender-differentiated nervousness is that men had natural resources of will-power which women lacked. In both medical and fictional texts, individual failure to exercise those powers is already underwritten with assumptions of abnormality. The narratives of Charlotte Brontë's Crimsworth and George Eliot's Latimer are framed within the debates of manliness which emerged from their respective contexts of gender, class, and economic organization.[33] In their different ways, these narratives register their assimilation of the construct of a medicalized definition of manliness and, at the same time, work to unsettle the assumptions which sustain them.

---

[32] Anne Brontë, *Agnes Grey* (1847), ed. by Angeline Goreau (Harmondsworth: Penguin, 1988), p. 65.
[33] Although *The Professor* was not published until 1857 (posthumously), it was her first novel, written in 1846 but rejected by her publishers, Smith, Elder & Co. during the intervening years.

HYPERSENSITIVE HEROES: *THE PROFESSOR* AND
'THE LIFTED VEIL'

Mid-century medicine was in a state of confusion over the problem of the hypersensitive male in a culture of manliness. William
Crimsworth, in Brontë's *The Professor*, and Latimer, in Eliot's
'The Lifted Veil', each present narratives of nervous sensibility
which call attention to the ambiguous and conflicting interpretations of normal and pathological experience. To different
degrees, and with varying levels of conscious reflection, their
narratives of 'self' are rather articulations of a pathological
'other' to the more robust and extrovert representatives of the
masculinist culture. Both have their beginnings in a profound
and affecting sense of isolation and marginalization from the
familial, class, and gender structures which underpin coherent
identity within their respective worlds of manufacturing and
finance. But where Crimsworth embarks upon a recuperative,
self-styled progress towards his own version of mature and
responsible manhood, Latimer persists in his constitutional
debility by endlessly reiterating the incompatibility of his supernatural power with the dictates of manly bourgeois realism
against which it is constantly measured.

Crimsworth's story is an autobiographical account of a man's
ascent from a position of class uncertainty and personal anxiety
to one of social, sexual, and psychological control.[34] My interest in this narrative is focused not so much on the story of that
rise or on the means by which it is achieved, rather, it is in
Brontë's representation of her hero as an anomaly in a cult of
masculinity which had been shaped and validated in no small
measure by medical science. Disadvantaged by his physical inferiority and position in the family, Crimsworth has to strive to
make his own way in the world and begins in the humble post
of second clerk in the mill owned by his older brother. In the
course of time, he moves to Belgium, becomes a schoolmaster,

---

[34] For a detailed study which locates Crimsworth's progress to social betterment
through a regime of self-regulation and control squarely in the light of Charlotte
Brontë's engagement with Victorian psychology, see Sally Shuttleworth, *Charlotte
Brontë and Victorian Psychology* (Cambridge: Cambridge University Press, 1996),
chapter 7.

acquires his own school, and, eventually, a wife and child. But far from being a pleasant, satisfying tale of success, it is one in which events and relationships are marked at every turn with antipathy and confrontation. It is true, as modern critics have pointed out, that the Victorian philosophy of 'self-help' is central to Crimsworth's progress towards integrated masculine identity.[35] But this is not to argue for Brontë's unequivocal endorsement of the principles and properties of that identity. On the contrary, the narrative is continually interrupted with ambivalences towards, and displacements of, the gendered, hier-archized models by which medical science sought to clarify the boundary between health and disease, and between normal and deviant functioning.

George Eliot's 'The Lifted Veil' is equally challenging of the cultural criteria by which medical science sought to separate and gender mental and physical organization in the mid-century period. Written in 1859, it tells the story, again in the form of a first-person narrative, of Latimer, who, when a young man, recovers from a fever to find that he has developed an extraor-dinary sensitivity. This sensitivity manifests itself in an ability both to see into the minds of others and to predict the future—including the time and manner of his own death. Clairvoyant power turns out to be a dubious blessing and the entire work is suffused with an air of oppressiveness and misery. [36] The concerns of the publisher, John Blackwood, about a tale which the author herself described as a *'jeu de melancolie'* or 'a slight story of an outré kind' were not lessened by the fact that the story culminates in a macabre scene depicting a medical exper-iment to revive a dead patient with a blood transfusion.[37] Far

---

[35] For example, see Heather Glen's introduction to the edition and Shuttleworth in the work cited above. The credo of 'self-help' was epitomized in the work of Samuel Smiles. Although the book *Self-Help* did not appear until 1859, Brontë was familiar with Smiles's preaching through local newspaper reports of his Leeds lectures.

[36] 'The Lifted Veil' was first published in *Blackwood's Magazine*, 86 (1859), 24–48. It was unsigned and unattributed.

[37] See Eliot's correspondence with John Blackwood in *The George Eliot Letters*, ed. by Gordon S. Haight, 9 vols. (London: Oxford University Press, 1954–78), iii. p. 41. Eliot's regard for the work and her conviction as to its significance can be ascertained from her refusal to compromise by removing the offending scene or to permit Blackwood to include it in a series of tales by various writers in 1873. *Letters*, v. p. 80.

from being a 'slight story' in the Eliot canon, and one which its contemporary critics, at best, politely passed over, 'The Lifted Veil' raises important questions about the cultural constructedness of the parameters of health and disease, and about the endlessly shifting contours of gender definition as the social, political, and economic needs of a particular culture drive the formation and modification of its models of normality.

In both of these texts, the protagonists are presented from the start as outcasts, marginalized by their peculiar sensitivities from the kind of unquestioning toughness and vigour which denoted the norm of manliness. Their position is one of powerlessness and, in psychological as well as social terms, closely allied to the feminine. Early in the narratives, both men register their subordination in terms of physical inferiority which is subsequently counterbalanced by their claims to mental superiority. We are told how each compares unfavourably in the manliness stakes with their elder brothers. Latimer's brother Alfred, a 'handsome self-confident man' is taller, stronger, more robust, well able to cope with the rigours, the 'rough experience' of Eton, and naturally fitted to be his father's 'representative and successor' in the tough, competitive world of banking and finance. Latimer is more instinctively drawn to his one friend and fellow student, Charles Meunier, who, although a brilliant scientist, is a social misfit, an object of pity and derision on account of the fact that he is 'poor and ugly', and therefore equally defective as a man.[38]

Similarly, Edward Crimsworth is presented as a fine specimen of English manhood with a 'robust frame' and 'athletic proportions'. Scrutinizing Edward, and then his own reflection in the mirror, William observes:

I looked at him: I measured his robust frame and powerful proportions; I saw my own reflection in the mirror over the mantelpiece; I amused myself with comparing the two pictures. In fact I resembled him, though I was not so handsome; my features were less regular; I had a darker eye, and a broader brow—in form I was greatly inferior—thinner, slighter, not so tall. As an animal, Edward excelled

[38] George Eliot, 'The Lifted Veil' (1859), ed. by Helen Small (Oxford: Oxford University Press, 1999), pp. 14, 8. Subsequent references to this edition will be given in the text.

me far; should he prove as paramount in mind as in person I must be a slave—for I must expect from him no lion-like generosity to one weaker than himself; his cold, avaricious eye, his stern, forbidding manner told me he would not spare. Had I then force of mind to cope with him? I did not know; I had never been tried.[39]

Crimsworth's suggestion that a correspondence between physical health and strength of will cannot be taken to be a reflection of moral worth draws attention to the confusions and shifts in the standard attributes of masculinity which, by mid-century, had moved away from the gentle moral manliness resonant of late Georgian sensibility. Although one must be cautious about attributing a characterizing uniformity to entire historical periods, there was, during the early decades of the nineteenth century, a perceptible change in a middle-class culture which fashioned sensitivity and delicacy as marks of civilized refinement to one in which nervousness was seen as an outward sign of latent mental disease. A perceived requirement for a more visibly vigorous manhood prompted the anxious scrutiny of physical features for their alleged indications of moral and psychological status.[40] If mid-century taste favoured a more muscular manliness, the ideal, represented here by Edward, is contested by Crimsworth's questioning of the seamless correspondence between manly vigour and moral rectitude. Both Brontë and Eliot challenge the conjunction of physical and moral supremacy when their womanish heroes claim for themselves the moral high ground. In autobiographies which implicitly disparage the brawny stalwartness that defines and sustains the bourgeois ideal of manliness, it is the feeble body that is posited as the index of high-mindedness.[41] Eliot, as we

---

[39] Charlotte Brontë, *The Professor* (1857), ed. by Heather Glen (Harmondsworth: Penguin, 1989), p. 49. Subsequent references to this edition will be given in the text.

[40] Sally Shuttleworth argues that knowledge of Brontë's fascination with the quasi-science of phrenology is crucial to the understanding of the force of the idea of the body's legibility. Unlike physiognomy, phrenology required very specialized expertise to interpret the meanings of individual cranial variations. It becomes important, therefore, to Crimsworth's self-validation as a man of superior worth to be possessed of the reading and interpretative skills which put him in a position of knowledge and power over and above his associates. *Charlotte Brontë and Victorian Psychology*, p. 128.

[41] The analogy between the attenuated body and high-mindedness was a familiar one, though disputed even at the height of the so-called cult of sensibility. James

shall see, complicates Latimer's claim to mental and moral superiority by compounding the mind/body equation with scientific theories about limited energy resources. But in Crimsworth's case, the dynamic shift from physical enfeeblement to moral strength gives credence to the systematic rejection of the world of industry and commerce in favour of that of the intellectual. His often overbearing self-righteousness is, in contrast to Latimer's self-disgust, in part, and paradoxically, a measure of his success in the production stakes. Brontë's novel, in this respect, presents an alternative route, if not to integration into the dominant masculine economy, at least to fulfilment of a perceived duty of production (in his case, the production and dissemination of knowledge) and reproduction (through continuation of the bourgeois family).

Reading *The Professor* as a narrative of maturation from emotionally alienated child to self-satisfied patriarch, it is impossible to ignore its uneasy and often disturbing sexuality. Finding expression through a metaphoric language of demons, of tyranny, and of haunting spectres, Crimsworth's burgeoning sexuality is communicated as a pathological process in which he has close correspondences with Latimer and with the morbidly introspective preoccupation with the body that was symptomatic of hypochondriasis. The tiresome, self-congratulatory resistance to the sexual and sensual indulgences of the more robust specimens of manhood is consistent with ideas of self-restraint which set the tone of the early-century ideal of moral manliness. But the collapse into an illness characterized by scarcely veiled sexual fantasies draws attention to the matter of repressed male sexuality and the self-vigilance necessitated by an increasingly vociferous rhetoric of male health and disease. Around mid-century, theories of male health were obsessively focused on sexual economy. Locating the key to a healthy economy in the conservation

---

Boswell had reflected on the fashionable notion: '*We Hypochondriacks* may . . . console ourselves in the hour of gloomy distress, by thinking that our sufferings mark our superiority'. He goes on, however, to question the validity of a proposition which ignores both the real misery of hypochondria and the wide range of its victims, from 'men of remarkable excellence' to 'as coarse mortals; nay, as silly creatures as ever appeared upon earth'. See *Boswell's Column: Being his Seventy Contributions to* THE LONDON MAGAZINE *under the Pseudonym* THE HYPOCHONDRIACK *from 1777 to 1783 here First Printed in Book Form in England*, ed. by Margery Bailey (London: William Kimber, 1951), pp. 42–3.

of vital resources, Victorian discourses on male sexuality became anxiously preoccupied with excess. Wilkie Collins's representation of Frederick Fairlie, to which I have already referred, plays on readers' familiarity with these very issues in 1860 when the self-obsessed recluse expresses his abhorrence of secretions other than those sufficiently removed from real life by 'the refining processes of Art' as to make them aesthetically appealing. 'I can understand', he explains in his Narrative at the point when his valet, Louis, admits Lady Glyde's tearful and perspiring maid, 'that a secretion may be healthy or unhealthy, but I cannot see the interest of a secretion from a sentimental point of view. Perhaps my own secretions being all wrong together, I am a little prejudiced on the subject' (347–8). Tears and perspiration are associated in his mind with the excesses of low-class persons unable to exercise due control over their emotions but, at the same time, secretions of any kind are rather too close for comfort to a man constantly at the mercy of his own bad humours.

Recent criticism has examined the deliberations on conservation and excess in relation to broader ideological concerns about male health and education. The opinions of medical men like William Acton, David Skae, and Henry Maudsley on the parameters of 'normal' and 'dysfunctional' sexual behaviour carried weight at a time when the new wealthy middle class sought to validate a set of educational practices on behalf of its sons. What were designated as the 'natural' excesses of young males were to be sublimated via compulsory physical activities in public and proprietary schools and thereafter channelled into production (of the nation's wealth) and reproduction (in the context of middle-class marriage).[42] It is true that many of the more lurid predictions as to the consequences of 'excess' were later dismissed by other doctors who expressed doubts about much that had passed for proven scientific fact. Thus, when

---

[42] See especially Ed Cohen, *Talk on the Wilde Side: Toward a Genealogy of a Discourse on Male Sexualities* (London: Routledge, 1993), pp. 35–68, for a detailed reading of the way in which a middle-class ideal of healthy manliness shaped male education in the nineteenth century. The forgotten writings of William Acton were brought to the attention of modern scholars by Steven Marcus in *The Other Victorians: A Study of Sexuality and Pornography in Mid-Nineteenth-Century England* (New York: Basic Books, 1964).

James Paget wrote of the way in which many male patients had come to regard 'trivial maladies, or even some of the natural events, in their sexual organs with the unreasonable dread or gloom and watchfulness which are characteristic of hypochondriasis', he did so in order to remove the demon of incipient madness that haunted men labouring under the misery of ignorance, made worse by the unscientific advice literature on which some had foolishly relied.[43] Paget's views are for the most part liberal and compassionate. He was convinced of the need for better education for both men and women to alleviate their distress. But his efforts to dispel the myths and apprise sufferers of the physiological facts can have done little to settle the minds of men already weighed down by the struggle against fear and prejudice, when his assurances about healthy manhood carried with them a sombre counterpoint of moral warning. His paper, 'Sexual Hypochondriasis' (1870), uses language which seems discordant with the general tone of edification. For instance, having pronounced that masturbation does not warrant the exaggerated dreads which men associate with it because they have been 'fraudulently misinformed', he adds: 'I wish that I could say something worse of so nasty a practice; an uncleanliness, a filthiness forbidden by GOD, an unmanliness despised by men'.[44]

The influence of this ongoing contention about excess and moderation is perceptible in the personal narratives of both Brontë's and Eliot's heroes in the tense undercurrents of a sexual energy that is variously diverted or suppressed. Sexual desire, in both texts, is mediated, in the first instance, through a voyeuristic participation in the sexual relationships of the older brothers, a process which sublimates even as it heightens and prolongs the watcher's desire. Crimsworth devitalizes the 'good

---

[43] James Paget, 'Sexual Hypochondriasis' (1870), in Howard Marsh (ed.), *Clinical Lectures and Essays*, 2nd edn. (London: Longmans, Green, 1879), pp. 275–6. For a study of Paget's influence and significance, see M. Jeanne Peterson, 'Dr. Acton's Enemy: Medicine, Sex, and Society in Victorian England', *Victorian Studies*, 29 (1986), 569–90. Though Acton has been widely quoted to represent the 'official' Victorian medical view and to exemplify the profession's 'tyranny' over the sexual lives of men and women, in this article Peterson questions the extent to which his pronouncements on sexual and social matters had weight or influence during the period.

[44] 'Sexual Hypochondriasis', p. 292.

animal spirits' (45) he observes in his brother's wife by reinterpreting them as coquetry and thereafter treating them with contempt. Latimer's exposure to the sexual charms of his brother's fiancée, Bertha, is more extended and complexly articulated. A passion which threatens to run out of control is set in contrast to the impassivity of his 'firm, unbending father', who is described as an 'intensely orderly man, . . . one of those people who are always like themselves from day to day, who are uninfluenced by the weather, and neither know melancholy nor high spirits'. Lacking his father's powers of self-regulation, the son is daily affected by the most commonplace of sensations with 'mingled trepidation and delicious excitement' (5). His passion for Bertha is increased by her very mystery and, while despising her inane shallowness, he none the less conjures sexual fantasies around her. Each day in her presence becomes 'a delicious torment' (17). He is 'completely under her sway', and, as he 'trembled under her touch', he felt for her 'a wild, hell-braving joy' (20). On one level, the simultaneous excitement of infatuation and terror of foreboding which characterize Latimer's doomed relationship with Bertha confirm his psychological instability. But, in the broader context of his culture, such excess and inconsistency underline the emasculating consequences of losing control as well as signalling the perils of a virility that is not channelled into business activities or public affairs.

Latimer's chronic affliction and Crimsworth's acute and temporary hypochondria are both strategies against, and symptoms of, ideals of manliness. As Heather Glen has pointed out, there is a curious contradiction between Crimsworth's projected image as a self-assured, self-made man, and the interminable watchful anxiety which renders him ever a prey to hypochondria.[45] It is true that the morbid introversion symptomatic of hypochondria was quite out of keeping with the ethos of athletic, outgoing, intrepid, and doubt-free manliness. But the

---

[45] Heather Glen reads Brontë's portrayal of Crimsworth as a 'fictional example of a quite distinct and influential contemporary genre . . . the exemplary biography of the self-made man.' Her reading carefully positions Crimsworth's narrative between, on the one hand, its alignment with the Victorian 'self-help' philosophy and, on the other, its disturbing problematization of the simple tale of self-improvement. Introduction to *The Professor*, pp. 9–12 (p. 10).

collapse into nervous disease is itself an indication of the toll upon the bodies and the minds of men who were unable or unwilling to partake of, even less compete in, the dominant cult of masculinity. Indeed, Crimsworth himself locates both the historical and the immediate causes of his hypochondria within these terms. He attributes his susceptibility to his having, throughout his young life, 'many affections and few objects, glowing aspirations and gloomy prospects, strong desires and slender hopes' (253), while his present parlous state is explained as the reaction of overwrought nerves to the exhausted body's weakness.

Striking him shortly before his marriage with Frances, the attack of hypochondria figures as the point of collision where the driving energy of firm conviction implodes into a private agony of uncertainty. The malady, named by Brontë as 'Hypochondria', is figured as a visitation by a darkly unpredictable, but eminently physical, female intrusion into the private space of the cerebral, nervously sensitive, man. And yet, in spite of the cold terror of anticipated prostration, it is clear that the patient is not altogether unwilling to succumb. It seems evident from Brontë's depiction of the disorder, not only in the case of *The Professor*, but equally in *Villette*, for which *The Professor* is traditionally held to be a prototype, that the term 'hypochondria' denoted more than a mere anxiety about the body's health. This passage from *The Professor* is a graphic illustration of the early Victorian understanding that this was an illness closely related to, if not caused by, sexual anxiety and tension:

She [Hypochondria] had been my acquaintance, nay, my guest, once before in boyhood; I had entertained her at bed and board for a year; for that space of time I had her to myself in secret; she lay with me, she ate with me, she walked out with me, showing me nooks in woods, hollows in hills, where we could sit together, and where she could drop her drear veil over me, and so hide sky and sun, grass and green tree; taking me entirely to her death-cold bosom, and holding me with arms of bone. What tales she would tell me at such hours! What songs she would recite in my ears! How she would discourse to me of her own country—the grave—and again and again promise to conduct me there ere long; and, drawing me to the very brink of a black, sullen river, show me, on the other side, shores unequal with mound, monument, and tablet, standing up in a glimmer more hoary than moonlight. (253)⁴⁶

For the invalid this sickness is no retreat of the kind which might legitimate self-indulgence and afford a temporary refuge from the unrelenting demands of manly resolution and duty. There is no denying the horror of the 'drear veil' which descends upon the sufferer and severs all connection with a genial world. But its meanings are interwoven and strangely ambiguous. On the one hand, the greatest dread is of the interruption to progress which an attack of hypochondria necessarily entails. This was an aspect of the malady which James Boswell had likened to the torment of Tantalus, where an overwhelming languour kept all the objects of his desire visible but out of reach.⁴⁷ It would make sense to read Crimsworth's anguish about his enforced retreat in these terms. Unsurprised by the previous visitations of his hypochondria, he is bewildered by this present timing just when sexual and social fulfilment are within his grasp. Weak from lack of sustenance and sleep due to a 'sweet delirium' of anticipation of the time 'when my desires, folding wings, weary with long flight . . . nestled there, warm, content, under the caress of a soft hand' (254–5), Crimsworth's hypochondria is the 'dreadful tyranny' which 'kept her sway over me for that night and the next day, and eight succeeding days' (254), preventing him from realizing his heart's desire. And yet, on the other hand, we are told how, in spite of all these horrors, Crimsworth 'had gone about as usual all the time, and had said nothing to anybody of what I felt' (254). Such resolve is entirely consistent with the ethic of self-control which underpinned a masculinist economy. But Crimsworth's imperviousness may equally hark back to earlier constructions of a disease whose worst excesses are those which affect the imagination rather than the body. On this very point, Boswell had observed how 'men of business who are afflicted with Hypochondria, however dilatory and negligent they may be in their private

---

⁴⁶ A popular book by J. R. Brodie entitled *The Secret Companion, a Medical Essay on the Treatment of Hypochondriacal Affections: Nervous and Mental Debility* was frequently advertised in the local newspapers and was read by Charlotte Brontë. See Sally Shuttleworth, *Charlotte Brontë and Victorian Psychology*, p. 273, n. 23.
⁴⁷ *Boswell's Column*, p. 49.

concerns, are yet able to go tolerably through with what is to be done in the way of their profession'.[48]

That hypochondria brought torments which, by their very nature, were largely invisible to outside observers who notice only the sufferer's peculiarities of temperament was documented in the Brontës' medical manual, Thomas John Graham's *Popular Domestic Medicine* (1826). A catalogue of symptoms ranging from 'groundless apprehensions of personal danger' to 'irksomeness and weariness of life' and from 'peevishness and general malevolence' to 'a whimsical dislike of particular persons, places or things' strikes the reader as both indeterminately vague and yet, at the same time, indiscriminately applicable.[49] Read in the light of Graham's description, Crimsworth's narrative takes on a whole new dimension in the sense that hypochondria defines the type of person he is, as well as diagnosing a specific event. To contextualize this further, the very secrecy with which the condition must be borne lends credence to a narrative more broadly concerned with individual feelings of isolation from the sentiments and sympathies that seem to bind the rest of society. It may be that the tense and ambiguous explorations of sexual power relations in *The Professor* replicate Brontë's own confusion, as woman and author, in negotiating the divide between an 'official' male perspective and the establishment, however tentatively, of an immanent female consciousness, as Helene Moglen has argued.[50] In the ensuing conflicts between masculinity and femininity, domination and submission, internal emotional energy and seeming surface control, Crimsworth is, by turns, feminized and aggressively masculine. The passivity which he assigns to himself during the period at the mill, and in contrast to his more powerful, more masculine brother, later becomes interwoven with a confused, repressed sexuality and a desire for sexual mastery. In the passage quoted above, images of sexual and social dominance vie with those of the fear of initiation in a drama which enacts

[48] *Boswell's Column*, pp. 50–1.
[49] Cited by Heather Glen, *The Professor*, p. 311, n. 20.
[50] Helene Moglen, *Charlotte Brontë: The Self Conceived* (New York: W. W. Norton, 1976), p. 88.

a reassigning of fixed gender positions.[51] Ultimately, the episode of acute hypochondria which has baffled many critics as to its narrative significance works to indicate a shift in the disease classification of hypochondriasis from an exclusively male psychosomatic disorder to a general indeterminate dread surrounding sexual and social identity. Undeniably, a restless sexual anxiety lies at the heart of Crimsworth's (or Brontë's) description of hypochondria. With this disease, where the fear of pain is both cause and symptom, '[t]he mind', James Boswell wrote, 'is full of scorpions'.[52] But in so far as recovery from sickness conventionally marks the end of ambivalence and the beginning of self-knowledge, what follows does not bear this out. Crimsworth's development towards mature manhood is marred by an incorrigible streak of violence barely suppressed beneath his patronizing and authoritarian attitude towards his wife and son. Unlike other literary depictions of states of altered consciousness which are sometimes strategic in bringing about a psychic transformation, Crimsworth's hypochondria stands uneasily in the narratorial scheme. If, however, we interpret hypochondria in terms of a broader negative disposition, as I have suggested, it explains Crimsworth's feelings of alienation and antipathy which characterize all his relations with others. Read as a single event, it figures only the invalid's temporary disconnection from the stable norms of rational progress.

The episode is none the less remarkable for its challenging of traditional concepts of sexual identity and narrative voice. It plays across the gendered dichotomies of activity and passivity, domination and submission, strength and fragility, with a voice that is strangely androgynous and, at the same time, insistently sexual. The authorial ambivalence that is systemic in *The Professor* deconstructs the boundaries of male or female fears and feelings to reveal a common anxiety about sexual initiation and commitment, and a dread of failure in the struggle to control and contain the overweening forces of nature with the exercise of moral self-management. It could be argued that Brontë's incorporation of hypochondria has to do with a

---

[51] Helene Moglen's psychosexual reading of Brontë's work offers a useful analysis of these relationships.

[52] *Boswell's Column*, p. 321.

personal need to concretize in the nervous body a sense of the invasion of the boundaries of the self in a world perceived as threatening. But, perhaps equally, her conflation of gender ambivalence and overwhelming dread illuminates an important locus of slippage where a predominantly male neurosis is modified into a non-gendered depressive disorder. By the time Brontë came to write *Villette*, the demon Hypochondria again rears her head as a spectre haunting a particularly susceptible type of person. Here, the recognition of one nervous body by another cuts through the private boundaries of individual suffering to figure neurosis as a sign and symbol of a more generalized experience of cultural dislocation. Recognizing the 'type' by phreno-logically reading the brow, eyes, and mouth, Lucy Snowe scrutinizes the King of Labassecour in attendance at a concert in Villette:

There sat a silent sufferer—a nervous, melancholy man. Those eyes had looked on the visits of a certain ghost—had long waited the comings and goings of that strangest spectre, Hypochondria. . . . Hypochondria has that wont, to rise in the midst of thousands—dark as Doom, pale as Malady, and well nigh strong as Death. Her comrade and victim thinks to be happy one moment—'Not so,' says she; 'I come.' And she freezes the blood in his heart, and beclouds the light in his eye.[53]

The unpredictability of this invasion of the self by the 'other' is again a prominent feature of an affliction which is both companionate (to its chosen 'comrade') and noxious (to its 'victim'), dreaded and yet sought out.[54]

---

[53] Charlotte Brontë, *Villette* (1853), ed. by Margaret Smith and Herbert Rosengarten (Oxford: Oxford University Press, 1984; with intro. by Margaret Smith, 1990), p. 267.

[54] It is clear from Brontë's correspondence that she diagnosed herself as a sufferer from hypochondria and that, as Heather Glen points out, she regarded the condition as 'a real disease, not to be dismissed as merely imaginary'. Writing to her former employer Miss Wooler, shortly after completing *The Professor*, Charlotte Brontë sympathizes with a fellow sufferer, a Mr Thomas, who 'for ten years . . . has felt the tyranny of Hypochondria. . . . I endured it but a year—and assuredly I can never forget the concentrated anguish of certain insufferable moments and the heavy gloom of many living hours—besides the preternatural horror which seemed to clothe existence and Nature—and which made life a continual waking Nightmare— under such circumstances the morbid nerves can know neither peace nor enjoy-ment'. *The Professor*, pp. 311–12, n. 20.

It is on this dual level—that is, of a state at once dreaded and familiar, of an illness both literal and figurative—that Eliot speaks of Latimer's 'demon', the morbid condition of excessive consciousness. For Eliot's sufferer the disease is chronic and relieved only temporarily, whereas for Brontë's Crimsworth it is acute, and we are encouraged, despite the less than convincing portrait of Victorian family life, to hope that the 'cure' will be permanent. Neither Crimsworth nor his readers can be certain, however, since it is clear that the illness, and not the patient, is the master. Although he succeeds in concealing his torment from the public eye, he is powerless to remove it and must suffer in silence until such time as 'the evil spirit departed from me' (254). Significantly, both men are freed from their demonic possession by marriage. Thus, when Latimer is first married to Bertha he experiences, for the first time since before his illness, a period of untrammelled and untroubled social and sexual fulfilment as well as a freedom from the affliction of prevision. But the anodyne is as double-edged as it is short lived. The pleasure and relief that his marriage brings is cynically dismissed as the 'intoxicated callousness which came from the delights of a first passion' (30), a short-term placebo designed to beguile the psyche into imagining the body to be cured. Crimsworth's marriage is at one level the culmination and consummation of his efforts as the self-made man, a triumph of self-discipline over all the odds of upbringing and temperament. While the narrative thus endorses the credo of self-help and individualism, it nevertheless highlights a deeply problematic ambivalence about an ideology which revered the qualities of toughness and competitiveness in its men of action.

The ideal of manliness was not, any more than its female correlative the 'angel in the house', without its internal ambiguities. Crimsworth's narrative of progressive self-help is, as I have suggested, continually undercut with contradictions which challenge the very tenets upon which it is constructed. Latimer's autobiography addresses those contradictions more directly by subjecting the terms of opposition, such as health and disease, excess and control, masculinity and femininity, to explicit interrogation. Eliot's text is concerned not at all with a recuperative progression from alienation to integration but with exploring the systems of meaning that have defined the norms and the deviations in the first place. For Latimer, unlike Crimsworth, self-help is a pointless ethic since his life story is already imprisoned between the phrenological prognosis of deficient masculinity and the foreknowledge of the time and manner of his death. From such an unpromising beginning, he embarks upon a tale not of social and psychological recovery but of morbid acceptance of a lot for which he hollowly craves sympathy.

In a brief reference to 'The Lifted Veil' in his biography of Eliot, Gordon S. Haight highlights the text's morbid concerns when he more or less dismisses it as 'the account of a young man named Latimer, who is *cursed* with exceptional intelligence, *afflicted* with clairvoyance, *suffering* from "the miseries of true prevision" '.[55] 'The Lifted Veil' has become one of the most critically discussed of Eliot's works in recent years. Modern readers are struck by the extraordinary intellectual and imaginative force of its engagement with the contentious issues of phrenology, clairvoyance, mesmerism, physiological psychology, and experimental medicine; in other words, by the very aspects which early readers found unpalatable. Alongside these issues, the narrative raises important questions about the way in which knowledge and experience are evaluated in terms of gender. Playing across the indeterminate space between 'masculine' science, objectivity, rationality, resolution, and vigour on the one hand, and 'feminine' nature, sensitivity, susceptibility, irresolution, and debility on the other, Eliot's text investigates the reliability of the criteria according to which knowledge was customarily separated and categorized in the period. Throughout the narrative, scientific rationality is set against poetic sensibility, measured fact against impression, present reality against preternatural vision. This is not to argue, however, that a binary oppositional model of science and art is, in itself, the key to explain this text.[56] Rather, absolute difference dissolves into a gradation whereby seemingly incompatible views of the world are shown to be shades or degrees of one another. Latimer's diseased perception is described in language

---

[55] Gordon S. Haight, *George Eliot: A Biography* (Oxford: Oxford University Press, 1968) p. 296, emphases in original.
[56] See Terry Eagleton, 'Power and Knowledge in "The Lifted Veil" ', *Literature and History*, 9 (1983), 52–61.

which draws attention to its slippage from, or its superfluity in relation to, an implied norm. We are constantly reminded of an 'excess' of sensitivity, passion, imagination, susceptibility, and of 'superadded consciousness', and equally, of a 'deficiency' of physique, of social skills, and of the power of self-regulation. An idea of a sliding scale of normality may well have been in Eliot's mind in 1859. By the time she came to write *Daniel Deronda* in 1876, and possibly influenced by Claude Bernard's work on the proportional relation of disease to health, the concept of alienation as a disturbed or exaggerated form of normal perception was more securely formulated.[57]

But, like so much of Eliot's writing, 'The Lifted Veil' is interrogative of ideas and assumptions and cannot be reduced to a simple theoretical principle. Indeed, many of Latimer's more bizarre analyses are framed as questions as he wrestles with the logic of the simultaneous truth of seemingly contrary beliefs. Some of these are worked through systematically but become endlessly compounded: 'Was this a dream . . . was it the poet's nature in me . . . Was it that my illness had wrought some happy change in my organisation—. . .?' (9–10). There are those questions which seem always to beg others, such as Latimer's deliberation on his 'strange new power . . . But *was* it a power?' (12), and which work simultaneously to undermine, or to raise objections to, the self-consoling explanations of phenomena. Others, unanswerable in the particular, appeal to some external authority and ultimately to the reader: 'Are you unable to give me your sympathy—you who read this? Are you unable to imagine this double consciousness at work within me . . .?' (21), or a general system of belief: 'What are all our personal loves when we have been sharing in that supreme agony?' (31). Inasmuch as this last question is an appeal for sympathy, its certain failure is signalled in the rhetorical form of the question itself. Eliot's study of the hypochondriacal, morbidly introspective hero works within the cultural dichotomies of mind and body, health and disease, masculine and feminine, but the interrogative mode adopted by Latimer in the attempt to organize and order his experience

---

[57] Bernard's work on pathology and physiology was a major influence on the ideas of G. H. Lewes, whose copy of *Leçons sur la physiologie et la pathologie du système nerveux* (1858) is extensively annotated.

continually tests those dichotomies by blurring the boundaries between the rational and the intuitive interpretations of phenomena.

Latimer's faculty for seeing beyond the veil of the material and the immediate is represented as a form of mental alienation and explicitly set against the desires and concerns of healthy, middle-class manhood.[58] Knowledge that he acquires through the manifestations of his diseased imagination is constantly evaluated alongside that sanctioned by a more worldly minded, workplace pragmatism. One of the central interests in 'The Lifted Veil' is the status of the knowledges deriving from the competing experiences of subjective and objective conscious- ness, where the former is allied to hypochondriacal self-absorp- tion and the latter to manly regulation and control. Once again, the particulars of fictional representation are indicative of a broader cultural tradition by which knowledge is hierarchized according to the seemingly incompatible, and implicitly gendered, discourses of imaginative sympathy and scientific rationality. Indeed, the argument of 'The Lifted Veil' presup- poses an awareness of a model in which the rational male was authorized to read, reveal, explain, or readjust the disordered female organization. What is particularly striking in Eliot's novella is the alternate adoption and overturning of the estab- lished gendered criteria, a process which disrupts the one-way dynamic of power. By making Latimer both empowered to 'read' and subjected to be read, Eliot unsettles the hierarchies which sustain belief in the objective authority of masculinist science over the subjective outpourings of the unregulated nature.

For Latimer, the process of feminization is both implicit and explicit. In the first instance, his role is compromised even in the paradigmatic male capacity for diagnosis and prognosis when he is given the kind of prescient vision more usually associated with an aberrant imagination. In the second, his subjection to phrenology, the practice which claimed to reveal hidden traits,

---

[58] Though I agree with Kate Flint's reading of 'The Lifted Veil' as an 'interroga- tion of the limits of positivism', my reading differs in its consideration of Eliot's well-documented knowledge of physiological psychology in the light of contempo- rary ideas of manliness. See 'Blood, Bodies, and *The Lifted Veil*', *Nineteenth- Century Literature*, 51/4 (1997), 455–73 (p. 458).

predict propensities, and estimate moral capacities according to the external configuration of the skull, is more overtly feminizing.[59] Early in the narrative, Latimer recalls how the phrenologist, summoned by his anxious father, pronounced him deficient in the area of the brain which denotes physical strength, prowess, and steadfastness, yet ominously superfluous in the area of imagination. A remedial programme is designed to eliminate all trace of feminine sensitivity in order to promote more appropriate and useful scientific and practical skills. While he longs for tales of 'human deeds and human emotions' (6), he is crammed instead with the rules of zoology and botany, electricity and magnetism. It is not the business of a man, he is instructed, to indulge the senses or the imagination 'with wandering thoughts' of the aesthetic appeal of running streams. Rather, 'an improved man, as distinguished from an ignorant one, was a man who knew the reason why water ran down-hill' (7). The disciplinary division of knowledge into scientific rationality and literary imagination has a venerable history of gender differentiation and one to which George Henry Lewes himself had been shown to subscribe. In his article 'The Lady Novelists', he had argued for the rightful place of women in literature very specifically on the grounds that their emotional lives fitted them for the expression of human experience and not for the strict formality of philosophy or science. He affirmed it a general rule that 'the Masculine mind is characterized by the predominance of the intellect, and the Feminine by the predominance of the emotions. According to this rough division', he continued, 'the regions of philosophy would be assigned to men, those of literature to women'.[60]

Ideas about the unsuitability of certain kinds of literature in the education of young men went hand in hand with fears of the unregulated nature and the perils of an imagination unchecked. The complex, and often contradictory, pronouncements on the

[59] Eliot's own engagement with phrenology is well known. B. M. Gray connects her interest with her friendship with Charles and Cara Bray. Eliot (then Marian Evans) exchanged letters with the phrenologist George Combe. See 'Pseudoscience and George Eliot's "The Lifted Veil" ', *Nineteeth-Century Fiction*, 36 (1982), 407–23.

[60] G. H. Lewes, 'The Lady Novelists', *Westminster Review*, o.s. 58 (1852), 129–41 (pp. 131–2).

subject of young male sexuality in a culture which was fast adjusting to a hitherto unprecedented level of medical intervention in all aspects of familial, economic, and national activity spawned a variety of 'solutions' through containment, sublimation, or displacement which, to some degree, invented the problems they sought to resolve. Doctors became spokesmen on education and social organization and, for reasons more political and economic than medical, imported the polarized models of manly vigour and irresolute effeminacy into educational and social policy. Much that passed for informed authority served only to reinforce ready-made gender distinctions, so that opinions on the emasculating effects of a poetic sensibility were strengthened by assumptions about the disciplinary divisions of science and literature. Two decades after 'The Lifted Veil', a writer in the *Westminster Review* was advocating a curriculum that 'would be solely scientific, would be the bare skeletons of abstract thought, scraped clean of every trace of living passion. And it is a well-proved fact that the scientific study of natural objects sometimes has a positive tendency to deaden our capacity for their poetical appreciation.'[61] This severe prescription has echoes of the salutary lesson meted out to Latimer, whose craving for classical literature must be satisfied in secret. When he confesses to reading 'Plutarch, and Shakespeare, and Don Quixote by the sly' (6), the recognition of the need for concealment is a defiance of the cultural standard of moral manliness and, paradoxically, an acceptance of the pathogenic, feminizing implications of the imaginative disposition.

Latimer's self-deprecating comments about his fragility and femininity, and his remarks on what was deemed a proper education for an English gentleman, are quite explicit and are presented in the light of the prevailing norms of English manliness. A delicate, tremulous child, Latimer tells us that he was 'held to have a sort of half-womanish, half-ghostly beauty' (14). He presents himself as a 'fragile, nervous, ineffectual self' using terms of reference more familiar in the framing of femininity:

---

[61] 'An Unrecognised Element in our Educational Systems', *Westminster Review*, n.s. 56 (1879), 197–210 (p. 207). The article is a recommendation for the teaching of the physiology of sex in schools—radical enough in 1879. But its fundamental premiss is that imagination is injurious to the psychological stability of young men and should be actively discouraged in their education.

But I thoroughly disliked my own *physique*, and nothing but the belief that it was a condition of poetic genius would have reconciled me to it. That brief hope was quite fled, and I saw in my face now nothing but the stamp of a morbid organisation, framed for passive suffering— too feeble for the sublime resistance of poetic production.   (14)

With this pitiful self-assessment, Latimer defines his weakness in both gender and economic terms. His enfeeblement, passivity, and morbid organization classify his condition within the language of female pathology. Although gifted with the sensi- tivity of the poet, he lacks the stamina for poetic production, an attribute which would have made him more acceptable to a bourgeois masculine economy. With no outlet for expression, his poetic sensibility atrophies into 'dumb passion' (7), a term which calls to mind a standard designation of womanhood as innately passionate and emotional, but crushed into mute subjection by the requirements of social respectability. At the same time, these unpropitious attributes are the particular bane of the second son whose prospects are insecure unless he can be harnessed to the productive imperative demanded by the new economic force. The division of individual propensity into scientific rationality and poetic sensibility resurfaces throughout the century in a variety of discourses. Henry Maudsley, for instance, considered he was simply facing facts when he dismissed John Conolly's poetry as 'slight poetical effusions'. If he had chosen to be a literary man rather than a physician, he continues, damning with faint praise, he would no doubt have excelled himself in 'light and easy versification'.[62] In both Maudsley's memoir and Eliot's fiction, the imaginative, literary disposition is culturally under-valued when judged by the stan- dards of a scientific and business economic order. By the same token, the male possessor of such a disposition is relegated to the feminine condition of feeble inconsequence.

When measured against the self-controlled objectivity of Victorian prescriptions of manliness, the subjective outpouring of pent-up feeling and fretful uncertainty is irretrievably aberrant, beyond the realms of reason and coherence. Vacillating between the miseries of imagination and the stultifying positivism of science, the story, in many respects, confounds interpretation.

[62] 'Memoir of the Late John Conolly, M.D.', p. 173.

On the one hand, the introspective, self-absorbed, hypochondriacal account of experience is, by the standards of Victorian manliness, pathological. And yet, Latimer's previsionary power, which exceeds the boundaries of private preoccupation and indeed the limits of normal human perception, is also portrayed as an affliction. Manifesting itself on two levels—namely his 'exasperating insight' (25) into others' thoughts and his prevision of future misery—it becomes a double curse. Problematically again, Latimer undertakes a task of self-narrativization which struggles at every turn to harness fugitive sensations and impressions to the scientific methodologies of hypothesis, experiment, analysis, and elimination. But the process of rational enquiry breaks down in the attempt to fix and objectify knowledge that is already doubly mediated, once through a form of mental aberration (clairvoyance), and again through memory (autobiographical recollections). Unlike Crimsworth, who endeavours to offset the deficiencies in manly attributes by promoting the supremacy of insight and sensitivity in assisting his passage to self-worth, Latimer insistently presses his affliction into the service of his already doomed, because self-centred, appeals for sympathy. Accordingly, 'The Lifted Veil' communicates the confessions of a man who, in his own words, has 'never fully unbosomed myself to any human being' (4) and who now yearns to exorcize the demon of insight and restore the commonplace attributes of manly pragmatism. As narrator, he cannot be trusted to distinguish between external reality and internal impression. Consequently, his autobiography plies an uncertain and discontinuous course in uncharted terrain, slipping imperceptibly between the record of experience he is anxious to complete before his imminent death, and an absurd and fanciful fiction whose origins lie in the creative impulse of the nervously susceptible mind.

Neat divisions between body and mind, health and disease, waking and dreaming, are variously eroded and crossed. If imagination and hypersensitivity to the incorporeal are construed as the morbid properties of the disordered mind, the authenticity of Latimer's narrative as a record of experience is cast into doubt. Alarmed by this possibility, he weighs the alternatives in the vain hope of establishing whether extrasensory perception was a desirable, power-conferring gift, or merely the 'unhealthy activity' of the hypochondriacal constitution: 'This strange new power had manifested itself again. . . . But *was* it a power? Might it not rather be a disease—a sort of intermittent delirium, concentrating my energy of brain into moments of unhealthy activity, and leaving my saner hours all the more barren?' (12, emphasis in original). He asks himself this question when, in the immediate aftermath of his first sighting of Bertha in the company of his father and a neighbour, Mrs Filmore, he is horrified to suspect that their presence might be a figment of his diseased imagination, a spectral vision indicating either a recurrence of his preternatural power or the onset of more intractable nervous disease. It is not insignificant that Latimer's first experience of insight into a realm beyond the material present occurs in the twilight world of fevered sickness as he drifts between levels of consciousness. When, subsequently, in yet another appeal for sympathy, he asks those who will read his story in the future to 'imagine this double consciousness at work within me, flowing on like two parallel streams that never mingle their waters and blend into a common hue' (21), the allusion to two separate modes of perception—the one firmly grounded in present reality, and the other linked to sense impressions originating in the unreality of a dreaming or hallucinatory state—is revealing of Eliot's acquaintance with contemporary neurology. Her friend and sometime consultant, Henry Holland, was of the opinion that health depended upon the symmetry of the two halves of the brain and, by extension, double consciousness could only indicate damage to the nervous connections.[63] In cases of 'mental derangement, as well as in some cases of hysteria which border upon it', he writes:

'[T]here appear, as it were, to be two distinct minds: one tending to correct by more just perceptions, feelings, and volitions, the aberrations of the other. . . . The cases just mentioned come under the description of what has been termed *double consciousness*; where the mind passes by alternation from one state to another, each having the perception of external impressions and appropriate trains of thought,

---

[63] Henry Holland was a Fellow of the Royal College of Physicians, Physician-Extraordinary to the Queen, and Physician-Ordinary to his Royal Highness Prince Albert. The third edition of his book, *Medical Notes and Reflections* (1855) was in Eliot's and Lewes's library, inscribed 'G. H. Lewes Esq. With the Author's best regards'.

but not linked together by the ordinary gradations, or by mutual memory.[64]

Sufferers of functional nervous disorders were thought to experience 'a double series of sensations; the real and unreal objects of sense impressing the individual so far simultaneously that the judgement and acts of mind are disordered' in such a way that the normal parameters of space, time, of mind and matter, of reality and imagination, become hopelessly distorted.[65]

In medical and fictional accounts of what Eliot calls 'super-added consciousness', the experience of perceiving beyond the veil of present material reality is routinely linked to episodes of illness. There are precedents, as Helen Small explains, for Eliot's use of the image of the veil as a film or curtain between life and death, or between knowledge/truth and ignorance, and for the association of seeing beyond the veil with horror and regret.[66] Latimer's somewhat tantalizing question as to whether the healthy body is the 'dull obstruction' (10) limiting human perception was one to which Brontë's Crimsworth knew the answer. For, while he laments that '[m]an is ever clogged with his mortality', he nevertheless recognizes that the unearthly rush of sound and 'the sensation of chill anguish accompanying it [which] many would have regarded as supernatural' (252–3), are signs and symptoms of nervous hypochondria. Scientists, as well as novelists, were eager to respond to the challenging questions arising from seeming supernatural experiences and to subject phenomena such as clairvoyance and mesmerism to scientific scrutiny. In 1851, the *Westminster Review* contributed to the debate about the scope and limits of human perception when, under the heading 'Electro-biology', a reviewer deplored the present public fascination with these pseudo-sciences and referred the more circumspect reader to the physiological or practical explanations offered by men of science.[67] Astonished by the gullibility of believers in this 'new art (science would be

---

[64] *Chapters on Mental Physiology*, 2nd edn. (London: Longman, Brown, Green, Longmans, and Roberts, 1858), pp. 196, 198, emphasis in original. This book formed part of an earlier edition of *Medical Notes and Reflections*, but was enlarged and published separately in 1852.

[65] *Chapters on Mental Physiology*, p. 196.

[66] 'The Lifted Veil', p. 88, n. 1.

[67] *Westminster Review*, 55 (1851), 312–28. The article reviews three works: J. H.

a misnomer)', the writer contends that no original knowledge can proceed from the revelations of individuals temporarily alienated from their immediate surroundings. 'The laws of suggestion', he writes, explain all this nonsense—as they explain too the phenomenon of clairvoyance:

There is nothing incredible in the statement of somnambulists predicting the hour of their sleeping or waking, nor in the dying foretelling the precise time of their decease. These are simply cases in which the mind, under the influence of a strong impression, *and acting upon a feeble physical organization,* has the power of fulfilling its own prophecy.[68]

Undoubtedly, this sceptic would have made short shrift of Latimer's advance knowledge of the time and manner of his death. When scientifically analysed, the so-called premonitory revelations can all be traced back to a direct external source such as another individual, a newspaper, or even by questions so framed as to contain the answer required. The very word 'clairvoyance' is a misnomer, he argues. 'Indeed, *clairvoyance,* instead of being clear-sightedness, is about the obscurest kind of vision, and most useless, that a human being can possess; for there is no well-authenticated case of a person discovering by it a single fact which it was of the slightest importance for him to know.' All the 'actions and predictions of the susceptible subject', he continues, 'are governed by past impressions, excepting those which may be communicated at the moment, by the partial action of any half-wakened sense'.[69] While this reasoning seems entirely convincing, its hasty dismissal of the way in which the alienated mind simply fulfils its own prophecy leaves much to be explained, not least the underlying assumption of a correlation between the impressionable mind and the feeble body. In an early, but influential, study of hypochondriasis, John Reid had included the phenomenon of accurate prediction of one's own death in a list of some of the more puzzling effects of fear, depression, or resignation upon the

Bennett, *The Mesmeric Mania of 1851, with a Physiological Explanation of the Phenomena produced; Chambers Journal for March, 1851* (No. 371); J. W. Haddock, *Somnolism and Phycheism [sic]; or the Science of the Soul and the Phenomena of Nervation.*

[68] *Westminster Review,* p. 327, my emphasis.
[69] Ibid., p. 328, emphasis in original.

minds and bodies of individuals suffering from hypochondria-sis.[70] As the medical profession sought to ratify its clinical opin-ions about the relations of the body and mind in health and disease, it turned to the physical sciences for a hypothesis of energy exchange.

In the continuing struggle to validate his insight as knowl-edge, Latimer overturns the orthodox association of hallucina-tory revelation with the mind deranged by fever and ponders the idea that illness, by devitalizing the body, correspondingly fine-tunes the inner life:

Was it that my illness had wrought some happy change in my organi-sation—given a firmer tension to my nerves—carried off some dull obstruction? I had often read of such effects—in works of fiction at least. Nay; in genuine biographies I had read of the subtilising or exalt-ing influence of some diseases on the mental powers. Did not Novalis feel his inspiration intensified under the progress of consumption? (10)

It was not just in 'works of fiction' or 'biographies' that these effects had been described. Through the years, many doctors had endorsed popular testimony to a correspondence between mental intensity and physical infirmity, and produced quantities of evidence to support a specific connection between consump-tion and exalted mental powers. In the 1880s, James Crichton-Browne, for example, referred to that well-known phenomenon of 'the intellectual vivacity, which so often accompanies incipi-ent phthisis'.[71] Latimer's excitement at the prospect that his bodily enfeeblement may be more than compensated for by creative genius has some foundation in medical precedent. We are reminded also of Crimsworth's ascription of high-minded-ness, embracing both mental and moral supremacy, to the puny body. Elements of the suggested link between bodily inferiority and mental excellence with which the nervously constituted

---

[70] John Reid, *Essays on Hypochondriasis*. Reid writes: 'Predictions of death, whether supposed to be supernatural, or originating from human authority, have often, in consequence of the poisonous operation of fear, been punctually fulfilled'. He goes on to cite the well-attested case of Lord Littleton, who 'expired at the exact stroke of the clock which, in a dream or vision, he had been forewarned would be the signal of his departure', p. 33.

[71] James Crichton-Browne, 'Education and the Nervous System', in Malcolm Morris (ed.), *The Book of Health* (London: Cassell, 1884), pp. 269–380 (p. 314).

male consoled himself are again at work here as Latimer anxiously applies them to his own experience of heightened sensitivity. But, without proof that his creative power is infinitely renewable, the true nature of Latimer's resources cannot be substantiated, and the dynamic relations of body and mind remain open to question.

With the phenomenon of physical diminution and mental agility familiar to doctors, it is easy to see how many of them came to be persuaded by scientific theories from outside the field of medicine of a finite, and perhaps even non-renewable, source of energy. The theory of finite energy, which appealed to doctors and the public alike, was based on the first and second laws of thermodynamics. Work begun by Sadi Carnot in 1824 on the available energy in closed systems was further developed by physicists including Helmholz, Clausius, Thomson, and Maxwell, all of whom saw a potential in this theory for explaining energy loss at both individual and cosmic levels. Put simply, the second law, formulated at mid-century, states that all forms of energy can be converted into other forms although, in the process, heat, which can never be entirely harnessed, gradually absorbs other energies into itself. Over time, the processes and structures dependent upon energy for life are deprived as that energy dissipates into useless heat. The great fear was of a condition of entropy in which all available energy would be exhausted and the system it supported would then collapse.[72] In the transference of ideas between disciplines and discourses, writers were quick to contextualize explanatory models, however ingenious, into their own narrative and structural schemes.[73] The implications raised by the complex and uncertain dynamics of body and

[72] For a discussion of the currency of the laws of entropy in (late) nineteenth-century culture, see Peter A. Dale, 'Thomas Hardy and the Best Consummation Possible', in John Christie and Sally Shuttleworth (eds.), *Nature Transfigured: Science and Literature, 1700–1900* (Manchester: Manchester University Press, 1989), pp. 206–7. Theories of finite energy came to be widely invoked in socio-medical treatises throughout the latter half of the nineteenth century to bring scientific weight to bear upon ready-made beliefs and prejudices, most particularly over the question of mental exertion at the expense of physical health. They were declaimed with especial vehemence, as I argue in Chapter 4, in the decades following Darwin's *The Origin of Species* (1859) and *The Descent of Man* (1871) in the accumulating anxieties about physiological degeneration.

[73] The transference from physics to physiology came about largely through the medical interest in 'animal heat' or 'vitalism'. The physiologist William Benjamin

mind, health and disease, are wide-ranging. For Latimer, they lie at the root of his dilemma since he has no way of knowing whether his heightened mental activity is the balance of physical deficit or merely the manifestation of disease. In a more general sense, the idea of the body and mind operating in an inverse ratio of credit and deficit raises the possibility that the balance might be tipped by chemical, mechanical, or psychological means. Much of the scientific interest in the nervous system was focused on the boundaries of waking, sleeping, and dreaming, and on how far medical intervention might reveal the mechanism by which body and mind communicated across the mysterious borderland of consciousness.

Indeed, in a final scene, Charles Meunier carries out a pioneering operation on the corpse of the servant Mrs Archer, transfusing her with his own blood to restore her vital functions long enough for her to reveal to Latimer the murderous secret of Bertha's mind that his own insight and precognitive powers have failed to reveal.[74] Rallying briefly, Archer points the finger of accusation at her mistress and gasps: ' "You mean to poison your husband . . . the poison is in the black cabinet . . . I got it for you . . . you laughed at me, and told lies about me behind my back, to make me disgusting . . . because you were jealous . . . are you sorry . . . now?" ' (42). If Eliot's early critics regretted the association of this affecting *mise-en-scène* with a demonstrably promising talent, it might be remembered that the decade immediately following its first publication in *Blackwood's Magazine* was to witness an upsurge of sensationalism in novel writing. The gothic proportions of this tale's climax both register and interrogate anxieties which inspired and propelled many a sensation theme. They stretch the imagination beyond the entropic end of energy exchange and challenge the impermeability of the closed system. Sliding together the physical drama of the deathbed scene and the mystifying

Carpenter, who also had an interest in zoology and marine biology, was a prominent figure in its application. In addition to his influential textbooks of mental physiology, Carpenter wrote extensively on the wider social and philosophical implications of developments in medical knowledge.

74 Recent re-readings of this scene include Kate Flint, 'Blood, Bodies, and *The Lifted Veil*'; Richard Menke, 'Fiction as Vivisection: G. H. Lewes and George Eliot', *ELH*, 67/2 (2000), 617–53.

dynamism of mesmeric performance, the visual and narrative 'spectacle' calls into question the integrity of the boundaries of the self and speculates on the relationship between agency and suggestibility. The assisted retrieval of knowledge from beyond the grave, so to speak, casts the doctor in a parallel role to that of the medium. Meunier's theatre shares with the hypnotist's stage the power of eliciting secret or repressed knowledge and desires during states of bodily torpor, a phenomenon to which the more marginal branches of experimental science bore ample witness.[75] Less compelling perhaps, but still deserving of attention, is the way that the interventionist role of the physician also brings back into focus the question of a hierarchy of knowledge and of the power of male science over the unregulated female nature.

The disputed boundaries of the scientific, and the intuitive and sentient interpretation of phenomena are interrogated to the last. Meunier stands paralysed by a momentary flash of insight into aspects of human life that are irreducible to a scientific problem, while Latimer imagines the horrifying possibility that medical ingenuity may revive the consciousness but leave the body insensible. The will, frozen for ever in the balance of 'half-committed sins', between consciousness and a powerlessness to act, ever 'rising to', 'ready to act out', is prevented by the body's permanent paralysis (42). Such disturbing possibilities call to mind the mesmeric experiment carried out on the dying M. Valdemar in Edgar Allan Poe's story *The Facts in the Case of M. Valdemar*.[76] Here, too, science intervenes in the normal processes of death in an attempt to separate the mind from the body. Latimer's horror of an artificially prolonged consciousness after physical death has taken place has a justified precedent in the case of M. Valdemar, whose death is arrested for seven months while he is held in a mesmeric trance. Only when his mind is finally released from the hypnotic state does his body return to the

---

[75] Not surprisingly, the reports of mesmerists are rich in such testimonies. It is clear from Eliot's correspondence that she was well informed as to their claims. B. M. Gray has recorded that Eliot herself visited a mesmerist, William Ballantyne Hodgson, in Liverpool in July 1844. 'Pseudoscience and George Eliot's "The Lifted Veil" ', pp. 412–13.

[76] Edgar Allan Poe, *Poetry and Tales*, ed. by Patrick F. Quinn (New York: Literary Classics of the United States, 1984).

condition of a seven-month cadaver. In 'The Lifted Veil', the answer to Latimer's question: 'Might there not lie some remedy for *me*, too, in [Meunier's] science?' (38, emphasis in original) is both 'yes' and 'no'. By bringing Latimer truths from behind the veil, experimental science has saved him from a death he had not foreseen and left the way open for his own prophecy to be fulfilled. But on the problematic subject of the 'psychological relations of disease' (38), it remains ominously silent, and there is neither explanation nor cure in Meunier's 'large and susceptible mind' for the malady of unwished-for insight which returns whenever Latimer is forced to cease his wanderings and settle in one place. His 'dying struggle' with the heart disease 'angina pectoris' calls attention once again to the figuration of the nervous body in the ambiguous terrain between organic reality and psychological interpretation. Eliot's choice of 'angina pectoris' is significant, bearing in mind her familiarity with the revisions to the causal criteria of this disease through the midcentury period. In 1846, George Man Burrows, whose book of physiology G. H. Lewes possessed, set out to prove a direct connection between functional disorders of the brain and heart disease. The pathology seemed less clear in the 1870s when angina was held to be a nervous disease and, like hysteria with which it shared the symptom of constriction of the chest and throat, or 'globus hystericus', brought on by mental and emotional causes acting upon the nerves. Also called 'cardiac neurosis', angina was well known to end in sudden death.[77] Knowing that the agonies of suffocation characteristic of angina will seize him at any moment, Latimer's narrative ends with a powerful confirmation of the 'miseries of true prevision' even as it affirms the reality of somatic illness against the whole catalogue of morbid imaginings of the nervous hypochondriac.

---

[77] George Man Burrows, *On Disorders of the Cerebral Circulation and on the Connection Between Affections of the Brain and Diseases of the Heart* (London: Longman, Brown, Green, and Longmans, 1846), pp. 105–6. In a discussion of the work of Charles Handfield-Jones, Physician to St Mary's Hospital, W. F. Bynum refers to Handfield-Jones's book, *Studies on Functional Nervous Disorder*, in which he uses the phrase 'cardiac neurosis' to refer to cases of angina as a category of neurological disorder. See 'The Nervous Patient in Eighteenth-and Nineteenth-Century Britain: The Psychiatric Origins of British Neurology', in W. F. Bynum, Roy Porter, and Michael Shepherd (eds.), *The Anatomy of Madness: Essays in the History of Psychiatry*, 3 vols. (London: Tavistock Publications, 1985), i. pp. 89–102 (p. 95).

In the decades after mid-century, the search for physical causes for indeterminate complaints meant that doctors and the general public were quick to recognize the nerves as the mechanism by which mental disorders might be materialized in the body, perhaps even traced to physical lesions in the brain. The nature of the relationship between body and mind became increasingly the province of the nerve specialist, and yet the positivist convictions of neurologists were not sufficient, in the absence of scientific proof, to erase traditional, conjectural, intuitive, subjective, even supernatural, interpretations of conditions which straddled the psychosomatic borderline. Old prejudices and assumptions about gender distinctions, about strength of will, or lack of moral fibre, continued to flourish as physiologists and psychologists argued over the nebulous aetiology of illnesses whose manifested symptoms were only too painfully apparent. The stigma of effeminacy continued to discountenance those men who failed to exercise due discipline over their allegedly wayward imaginations or to channel their creative energies into practical pursuits. As Latimer testifies, 'the poet's sensibility that finds no vent but in silent tears' and shudders inwardly 'at the sound of harsh human tones' has no place in the changed world of the workplace. Fine sensibilities, once esteemed, now bring with them only a 'fatal solitude of soul in the society of one's fellow-men' (7). The egocentric narrations of hypochondria or diseased consciousness confirm the anomalous status of the hypersensitive man in a culture which favoured a vigorously outgoing contribution to the familial and national economy. On the other hand, the very idea of a subjective narrative of disorder, let alone one which was implicitly critical of the ideological determinants of disease specification and diagnosis, might be seen to question the integrity of a medical fraternity seeking to establish its professionalism through scientific objectivity. It was not until towards the end of the century and the advent of psychoanalysis that medical discourse adopted, in the case study, a form that approximated literary narrative.[78] Neither hypochondriasis nor hysteria disappeared

[78] Jan Goldstein makes the same observation in her study of the intersection of medical and literary discourse in nineteenth-century France. 'The Uses of Male Hysteria', pp. 137–8.

from medical textbooks but defining lines were continually re-drawn in order to include new symptoms purportedly arising from new social conditions. Once it could be convincingly argued that the nerves, like any other material structure or mechanism, could be worn out through strenuous use, then the causes of nervous collapse might be sought in overwork or trauma and not in the emotional or moral weakness frequently associated with women and femininely fragile men. The more fashionable mechanical analogy gave a new impetus to those seeking to re-establish clear boundaries between male and female forms of functional disorder, and between masculine men, whose hitherto inexplicable prostration could now be accounted for physiologically, and effeminate men, who could boast no such heroic excuse. But as more came to be understood about the workings of the nervous system in determining and regulating both mental and physical well-being, this was by no means automatically followed by a more sympathetic approach to nervously susceptible men. Developments in neurology seemed rather to open up new divisions between real and imag-inary disorders and to reinforce old ones between constitutional debility and occupational strain.

Working with and against the cultural criteria which pathol-ogized the hypersensitive man at a time of industrial and impe-rialist expansion, the literary texts discussed here reveal many of the contradictions and ambiguities which medical discourse masked. Female-authored narratives of male subjectivity are unsettling in themselves. Charlotte Brontë's portrait of Crimsworth is, in significant ways, in line with the principles and tenets which drove an orthodox masculinist culture towards its individualist goals. Her hero's triumph of self-disci-pline is achieved partly by his disturbing adoption and utiliza-tion of the aggressive tactics which he had earlier scorned. But at the same time, Brontë's narrative problematizes rather than sanctions the attributes of tough impassivity with which Crimsworth has to contend in the man's world. In 'The Lifted Veil', there is no mention of hysteria or hypochondria, but the language of Eliot's exposition of Latimer's 'morbid organisa-tion' is that which can be found in any number of contemporary medical texts where physicians routinely constructed their nervously ill male patients within a frame of female pathology or unmanly dread. At the same time, it is a language that harbours within its ambiguities the private anxieties about authorship and self-expression which haunted both Eliot and Brontë for much of their early fiction-writing careers.[79]

When, in bemoaning the ease with which written histories can compress years of misery and pain into a single sentence, Latimer muses: 'We learn *words* by rote, but not their meaning; *that* must be paid for with our life-blood, and printed in the subtle fibres of our nerves' (34, emphasis in original), he not only suggests a process whereby sensory impressions are assimilated into consciousness, but raises once again the biologistic assertion that the body must, in turn, pay the price for mental toil. As physicians strengthened the morbid connections between heightened perception, exaggerated sensitivity, and the diminished will-power observed in neuroses, the hypersensitive man lived in dread of being overtaken by imperceptible, but irresistible, forces which threatened, not from an external source, but more alarmingly, from inside the self.

[79] Eliot expressed her own 'morbid sensibility' with relation to the growing speculation as to the authorship of *Adam Bede* when she wrote to Charles Bray on 26 September, 1859. *The George Eliot Letters*, iii. p. 164.

CHAPTER THREE

The 'Unmapped Country': Physiology, Consciousness, and the Mysteries of the Inner Life

BASIL AND FICTIONS OF DELIRIUM

As some authors explored the effects of emotional distress, or of a sense of isolation and displacement upon the body, others turned their attention to the relationship between physiology and consciousness. This difference of focus reflects a mid-nineteenth century fascination with the nature of consciousness and with the scientific analysis of experiences such as dreaming, delirium, hallucination, and spectral illusion. New medical journals specializing in 'mental science' appeared and the subject of the workings of the mind in various states of awareness was regularly debated both in the weighty and more popular periodicals including *Household Words*, *Macmillan's Magazine*, the *Fortnightly Review*, the *Westminster Review*, and the *Quarterly Review*, as Jenny Bourne Taylor has shown.[1] Both Wilkie Collins and Charles Dickens actively participated in the debates through the forum of *Household Words*. In 1852, the year of the publication of *Basil*, an article appeared in Dickens's magazine confidently pronouncing that science was on the point of discovering 'new explanations' for all the mysteries of what Collins, in the novel, describes as 'the workings of the hidden life within us which we may experience but cannot explain'.[2]

---

[1] 'Obscure Recesses: Locating the Victorian Unconscious', in J. B. Bullen (ed.), *Writing and Victorianism* (New York: Longman, 1997), pp. 137–79.

[2] Wilkie Collins, *Basil* (1852), ed. by Dorothy Goldman (Oxford: Oxford University Press, 1990), p. 29. Subsequent references to this edition will be given in the text. See also Henry Morley, 'New Discoveries in Ghosts', *Household Words*, 95 (January, 1852), 403–6.

William Benjamin Carpenter, an eminent physiologist, devoted a chapter in *Principles of Human Physiology* (1853) to 'The Cerebrum, and its Functions' in which he set out to elucidate the very mysteries of consciousness in relation to the range of normal and morbid mental states which so intrigued Collins. Carpenter's designation of the term 'unconscious cerebration' for the continuous operations of the brain outside conscious awareness provided a model for formalizing the familiar but bewildering perceptual aberrations which occur in dreaming or delirious states.[3]

Collins's *Basil* and Dickens's *Great Expectations* and *Bleak House* are only three of the many literary texts in the period shortly after mid-century which make use of the altered consciousness experienced in delirium to examine concepts of identity away from the objects and events which fill normal waking life. As Basil, Pip, and Esther, respectively, enter realms in which the mind is active while voluntary control over the current of thought is totally relinquished, their narratives slip between the real and psychic worlds, confusing the boundaries which usually distinguish one from the other. The second part of the chapter turns to the period when mental science became more directly linked to physiology and neurology through the fast developing life sciences. In the years leading up to 1876, when George Eliot's *Daniel Deronda* was published, George Henry Lewes was researching the physiology of the nervous system for his *Problems of Life and Mind*. My focus on *Daniel Deronda*, and especially on Eliot's representation of Gwendolen Harleth, is indicative of the close similiarity of the kinds of questions posed by the scientist and the novelist as they conducted their own investigations into 'life and mind'. More than that, Eliot's study of the gradual dislocation of a young woman's consciousness from the social world she inhabits is one of the most subtle and sophisticated explorations of 'the workings of the hidden life within us' in nineteenth-century fiction.

[3] Carpenter used the term 'unconscious cerebration' in the fourth edition of *Principles of Human Physiology* (London: John Churchill, 1853), p. 819, but scientific theories about the workings of the brain below conscious levels had been in the public domain at least since the 1830s and both Collins and Dickens were aware of them. Another influential work on the physiology of consciousness was Thomas Laycock, *Mind and Brain: or, The Correlations of Consciousness and Organisation*, 2 vols. (Edinburgh: Sutherland and Knox, 1860).

One of the features of delirium which seemed to fire the imagination of fiction writers was its capacity for opening up areas of a patient's mental life of which he or she was otherwise quite unaware. Unsurprisingly, many people wanted to believe that these transportations to a world beyond the veil, as it were, privileged the dreamer with supernatural insights. Questions about unified selfhood and about the reliability of knowledge imparted to individuals during such states were fiercely debated, with some writers more convinced than others as to the scientific significance of dreaming experiences.[4] Henry Holland believed that the borderline states between waking consciousness and profound sleep, states which included dreaming and delirium, gave a 'continuity' to all the bewildering, discontinuous 'phenomena of our being'. Dreaming, he wrote, 'forms a passage' in which the mind is 'capable of recognizing those rapid and repeated changes by which it shifts to each side of the imaginary line'. Those 'strange aberrations of thought' which occur in the 'slumbering moments' are not wholly disconnected from the rational structures of waking consciousness, but are suggestive merely of altered perspectives and changed priorities.[5] Taken at face value, this kaleidoscopic theory of the dreaming process seems rather dismissive of the belief in special insight. But for medical scientists, the investigation of dreams and delirium held more challenges than simply that of finding analogies for dreaming experiences in the events of waking life. In what these states might reveal were far larger questions about the nature of the relationship between different levels of consciousness and, in turn, about the role of the brain and nervous system in moving from one level to another. Quite apart from the contested issue of whether dreams and delirium afforded the dreamer privileged insight, more basic questions about what is normal and what pathological in respect of individuals' semi-conscious experiences were, of course, central to the debates.[6] At one end

---

[4] Jenny Bourne Taylor discusses these and other questions in relation to Victorian conceptualizations and representations of the 'unconscious' in 'Obscure Recesses'.

[5] *Chapters on Mental Physiology*, pp. 4, 12. On the subject of premonitory dreams the scepticism of a commentator in the *Westminster Review*, 55 (1851) has already been noted in Chapter 2, n. 68.

[6] See Taylor, 'Obscure Recesses', pp. 142–3.

of the psychosomatic spectrum, delirium marks the point of crisis in the progress of diseases such as typhus or smallpox. In the absence of organic disease, on the other hand, visions, hallucinations, and trance-like waking dreams were frequently associated with moral or emotional derangement or seen as signs of incipient insanity. Medical science had to be interpretative as well as diagnostic. As the century progressed, the philosophical and metaphysical questions which these states of altered consciousness posed for psychology were increasingly rephrased as physiological and, more particularly, as neurological ones.

These were not questions, however, confined to medical circles. For novelists, the imaginative possibilities of the hidden powers in a mind released from the restraining inhibitions of full consciousness were infinitely utilizable. Fictional uses of delirium range in form from a simple narrative device to the paralysing crisis of identity, and in content between psychic transformation and somatic deterioration.[7] In some texts delirium is significant in marking a turn in the overall narrative, whilst in others it creates a liminal domain where the laws and codes which fix consciousness in the material present are temporarily suspended. As a narrative device, delirium enables revelations and transformations that would seem implausible in realist plot. Hidden structures of relations and connections between mental life and the material world become accessible through the unlikely agency of afflictions characterized by derangement of the faculties. The often startling visions and insights experienced by the delirious patient when released from the encumbrances of the objects of waking reality enable writers to explore the relationships between body and mind, health and morbidity, imagination and reality, remembrance and oblivion. Many doctors were willing to concede, like James Cowles

---

[7] Instances of this diversity might include Dickens's Eugene Wrayburn, whose delirium is unambiguously caused by the brutal attack on him by Bradley Headstone, but which also works figuratively as a punitive and corrective device. *Our Mutual Friend* (1864–5), ed. by Stephen Gill (Harmondsworth: Penguin, 1971), pp. 805–12. George Meredith's Lucy Feverel, on the other hand, suffers from brain fever brought on by emotional causes of sorrow and disappointment and which, unusually in fiction of this period, ends in her death. *The Ordeal of Richard Feverel*, new edn. (London: Chapman and Hall, 1894), pp. 468–72.

Prichard, that when the mind was 'thus drawn into itself' and no longer encumbered with 'the perception of surrounding objects', its seeming capacity for memory recall or creative composition left them continually astonished and baffled.[8] The mysterious landscapes of altered consciousness were fertile grounds where writers, medical and literary, could test the scope and limitations of human perception and challenge the familiar norms of unified selfhood.

Between the years 1850 and 1870, the period which included the decade of the sensation novel, many writers made tacit correspondences between the particular puzzles and paradoxes in medical and lay theories of delirium and more general anxieties about identity and self-control. To put this another way, vague notions about the psychological stability of the self, about coherence and continuity, and about the reliability of the impressions which secure individuals' sense of their own place in an interpretable external world, were made more explicit through the crisis of delirium. In some fiction, such as Mrs Henry Wood's *East Lynne*, for example, delirium functions at the simplest level of a narrative device, a mechanism for absorbing or imparting information while the character's controlling will is in temporary abeyance. When, in *East Lynne*, Isabel Carlyle overhears the gossip about the conjectured close relationship between her husband, Archibald, and Barbara Hare, much is made of the fact that she was just emerging from a state of 'half sleep, half wakeful delirium, which those who suffer from weakness and fever know only too well'.[9] As the gossipers continue with their predictions for the future, should Isabel die and Barbara Hare step into her shoes, the narrator explains how delirium renders the mind suggestible to the implantation of ideas which would make no impression upon the mind in a strong state of health. It is, of course, vital to the plot that Isabel is apprised of the details which sow the seeds in her mind of her husband's faithlessness, and it is her weakness, feverishness, and 'state of partial delirium' that allow those seeds to flourish.[10]

---

[8] *The Cyclopaedia of Practical Medicine*, ed. by J. Forbes, A. Tweedie, and J. Conolly, 4 vols. (London: Sherwood, Gilbert, Piper *et al.*, 1833–5), i. pp. 506–7.
[9] *East Lynne* (1861), ed. by Stevie Davies (London: Dent, 1984), p. 179.
[10] Ibid., p. 183.

While not wanting to overstate the coincidence of sensation-alism and delirium, there is a point to be made in that both represent breaks, disruptions in the stable norms of progressive development. The aberrant act or anomalous individual, char-acteristic of sensation themes, constitute disturbances in the seemingly calm surfaces of a moral and social order; similarly, the feverish wanderings of delirium introduce interruptions in the pattern of normal, waking life. Sally Shuttleworth has argued that sensation fiction, both in form and content, mounted an assault on bourgeois realism by violating the very codes of coherence and continuity which were necessary to support its models of social and psychological stability.[11] Writers exploited the contested aetiologies of disease which they found in medical knowledge in order to incorporate uncertainty and inconsistency into their narratives of physiological and psychological collapse. These 'feverish productions', as Margaret Oliphant labelled sensation novels, made use of discontinuity and defamiliarization to stimulate the reader into a state of excitement and perplexity about the unverifiability of authorized versions of normality and reality.[12] Delirium repli-cates the transient, paroxysmal, and unpredictable aspects of experience and so disrupts, both for characters and readers, the reassuringly logical progression towards self-knowledge and social betterment. That insertion of temporary or partial breaks in an individual's progress is an important feature of writing which seeks to challenge the consolatory paradigms of auton-omy, coherent identity, and a controlling will. When they included delirium in the lives of their characters, the novelists discussed here were aiming to explore the perplexing ontologi-cal questions which the phenomenon raises. This is not to deny the delirious patient his or her suffering and terror. The experi-ence for Collins's Basil was a 'frightful' exaggeration of sensa-tions and images concentrated into a phantasmagoric nightmare (169). Similarly, for Dickens's Esther, the remembrance of the endless toiling and torment leaves her afraid even to 'hint at' the

[11] See 'Preaching to the Nerves: Psychological Disorder in Sensation Fiction', in M. Benjamin (ed.), *A Question of Identity: Women, Science and Literature* (Newark, NJ: Rutgers University Press, 1993), pp. 192–244.
[12] [Margaret Oliphant], 'Sensation Novels', *Blackwood's Magazine*, 102 (1867), 257–80 (p. 275).

detail of her 'sick experiences' to any but fellow sufferers.[13]
Delirium harbours the uncanny in its seeming power to facili-
tate insights and mental processes alien to the rationality of
wakefulness whilst, at the same time and more disturbingly,
revealing aspects of the human mind which operate outside the
control of the will.

In our antibiotic fever-controlled medical culture, we have
little experience of the state of delirium, especially of febrile
delirium. It scarcely needs to be said that this was far from the
case in the nineteenth century, when the majority will have
observed, or have had personal experience of, the phenomenon
whose multiform manifestations gave rise to a variety of interpretations. James Cowles Prichard writes in the *Cyclopaedia of
Practical Medicine*:

> The term delirium has either been employed without design in a vague
> and indefinite manner, or it has been purposely used in a very compre-
> hensive sense, and made to include every mode and degree of mental
> disturbance, from the slight and difficultly-traced aberrations of the
> argumentative and almost rational monomaniac, to the muttering and
> dreamy stupor of a patient labouring under the delirium of typhoid
> fever. All the phases and varieties of mental alienation, whether degrees
> of melancholy or violent madness, the wild ravings of the drunkard
> and the intense reveries of the opium-eater, as well as the peculiar
> symptoms resulting from that oppressed and disturbed condition of
> the sensorium which exists in severe febrile complaints, are alike
> comprehended under the designation of delirium when thus exten-
> sively applied.[14]

In their representations of the brain-fevered protagonist, Basil,
and the delirious invalids, Pip and Esther, Collins and Dickens,
respectively, exploit the paradoxes of delirium to construct
narratives which reflect, modify, or amplify the observations
made in these remarks.

Wilkie Collins was no stranger to the developments in mental
science and, throughout a long writing career, his novels bear
witness to the shifting credibility of a number of theories,

[13] Charles Dickens, *Bleak House* (1853), ed. by Norman Page with intro. by J.
Hillis Miller (Harmondsworth: Penguin, 1971), p. 544. Subsequent references to
this edition will be given in the text.
[14] *The Cyclopaedia of Practical Medicine*, i. p. 506.

including associational psychology and 'unconscious cerebration'. It is not difficult to find images of associationism—the theory that the mind 'thinks' and makes sense of the world by making connections between one idea and another—in *Basil* or, indeed, in any of Collins's fictions. He was, however, continually researching and refining his ideas and, although it is not until 1879 that one of his fictional characters openly acknowledges that 'we think of something, consciously or unconsciously, in the daytime, and then reproduce it in a dream', it is clear that an understanding of the brain's continual activity of processing and storing at levels below conscious awareness is already in place in 1852.[15] In *Basil*, Collins makes use of the unconscious thought processes activated by delirium in ways which, in the light of Prichard's categories cited above, would come under the head of 'purposely used in a very comprehensive sense'. The whole gamut of physiological and psychological causes is brought under suspicion in a complex interweaving of nervous susceptibility, hypersensitivity, incipient madness, violence, and contagious association. As with Brontë's *The Professor* and Eliot's 'The Lifted Veil', the subject of Collins's narrative is the sensitive younger son of an upper middle-class family. Interesting comparisons are to be made with these texts in respect of the morbidly hypersensitive male, a figure whose representation, as I have already shown, was significantly shaped by mid-century notions of manliness. In Basil's case, youthful vulnerability, heightened sensitivity, burgeoning sexual curiosity, and morbid anxiety are mutually reinforcing elements in the production of 'a melancholic hovering on the brink of monomania'.[16] Introspective, fearful, and impressionable, his nervous sensitivity is registered in and on his attenuated body. Like Crimsworth and Latimer, Basil is the feebler brother of a more physically robust sibling, describing the bond between them as being 'so strangely compounded of my weakness and

---

[15] The remark is made by Mrs Farnaby in *The Fallen Leaves* (1879). For a reading of associationism in Collins's novels, see C. M. Tingle, 'Symptomatic Writings: Prefigurations of Freudian Theories and Models of the Mind in the Fiction of Sheridan Le Fanu, Wilkie Collins and George Eliot', unpublished Ph.D. thesis (University of Leeds, 2000).

[16] Jenny Bourne Taylor, *In The Secret Theatre of Home: Wilkie Collins, Sensation Narrative, and Nineteenth-Century Psychology* (London: Routledge, 1988), p. 74.

his strength; of my passive and of his active nature' (256). Incorporating both constitutional and environmental aspects of nervous pathology, the story of Basil's breakdown is a sensation-alized version of a young man's struggle towards coherent social identity and sexual maturity. Written as a first-person narrative, it tells the story of Basil's sudden obsession with a dark and allur-ing girl he sees on an omnibus. Margaret Sherwin, it turns out, is the daughter of a London linen-draper, and the unlikely courtship upon which the hero embarks takes Basil into an unfa-miliar suburban world of trade, new money, and values very different from his own. Spurred on by his desire for Margaret, Basil agrees to a 'marriage' which must remain both secret and unconsummated for a year. But on the eve of the day which is to end his waiting, Basil discovers the terrible truth of his betrothed's seduction by her father's clerk, Mannion. Crazed with shock and anger, Basil attacks Mannion, smashing his face into the newly granite-surfaced road and leaving him hideously disfigured. After wandering blindly around the streets for several hours, Basil collapses into unconsciousness and is returned to his father's house where brain fever sets in and he passes through a long trial of delirium. The different levels of consciousness draw him back through landscapes of experience in which his sensa-tions and impressions are replayed, but now force from him new interpretations of their meanings and significances.

The story leading up to Basil's breakdown is a feverish explo-ration of impressionability and obsession.[17] Throughout the hero's labyrinthine journey of social, emotional, and moral dislo-cation, the sense of fevered pursuit combined with nervous dread becomes amplified into a nightmare world in which trauma and terror dissolve the boundaries between the real and the imag-ined. The representation of Basil's psychosomatic sickness is indeed 'comprehensive', playing across documented medical

[17] Similarly, in Collins's short story 'Mad Monkton', also published in 1852, the onset of brain fever is directly related to the hero's disappointment in the failure of an obsessive quest. Although Alfred Monkton dies, however, it remains open to interpretation whether his death (following a brief recovery from fever) was the fulfilment of his morbid prophecy, a mere coincidence, or, indeed, whether the monomaniacal obsession terminating in his fever was itself a symptom of hereditary insanity. Unlike Basil, Monkton emerges from the brain fever with no recollection of the events which led up to it. *Mad Monkton and Other Stories*, ed. by Norman Page (Oxford: Oxford University Press, 1994).

reference and popular surmise. Basil's condition, of which, even at the height of its convulsive strength, he is partly aware, is diagnosed as a fever which 'had seized on my brain' (175). Brain fever, though a widely inclusive disorder, had the advantage of being perceived as 'real' and was immediately recognizable to a contemporary readership as physiological and, therefore, distinct from madness. Audrey Peterson's assessment of brain fever in fiction has shown how a disease that was almost always fatal in real life translates into a mechanism whereby the literary victim more usually survives to 'continue to function in the narrative' although altered irreversibly by the experience.[18] It is its unpredictability and indeterminacy, and, above all, its 'combination of emotional cause and physical effect', writes Peterson, that made brain fever such a compelling concept for the novelist.[19]

It was well known among patients and practitioners that psychological stress was a powerful determinant in instigating physiological symptoms. For some writers, however, such a readily identifiable causal connection, though implied, was not altogether the point. Charlotte Brontë, for example, whilst adamant that depression can lead on to physical illness, is at pains to emphasize the uncertainty about the dynamic relation of body and mind in contributing to disease. When, in *Villette*, she describes Lucy Snowe's prostration during the long vacation as a 'strange fever of the nerves and blood', it is the 'unknown anguish' of the 'nameless experience' which gives febrile delirium its capacity for heightening anxiety and for making the condition exacerbate the tensions which led up to it. As days and nights of 'peculiarly agonizing depression' turn to physical illness, the terror and desolation in Lucy's mind become indistinguishable from the imagined pain of an obstruction of the heart and blood. The agent of this morbid interaction is, she suspects, 'my "nervous system" '.[20] In *Basil*, the very uncertainty in which the

---

[18] Audrey C. Peterson, 'Brain Fever in Nineteenth-Century Literature: Fact and Fiction', *Victorian Studies*, 19 (1976), 445–64 (p. 449). Elizabeth Gaskell's Phillis Holman is an example of a brain fever sufferer who, like Basil, survives. *Cousin Phillis* (1864), ed. by Peter Keating (Harmondsworth: Penguin, 1976).

[19] 'Brain Fever in Nineteenth-Century Literature', p. 464.

[20] Charlotte Brontë, *Villette*, ed. by Margaret Smith and Herbert Rosengarten (Oxford: Oxford University Press, 1984; with intro. by Margaret Smith, 1990), pp. 197, 231.

causal criteria of fevers of the brain were shrouded plays into the hands of the sensation writer by compounding the sense of a nightmare world of indecipherable codes and mistaken impressions. Collins's fascinated curiosity about the relationship between the mind and the brain can be evidenced elsewhere in 1852, when he contributed articles entitled 'Magnetic Evenings at Home' to G. H. Lewes's journal, *The Leader*.[21] The articles raise a whole series of questions about the mysterious processes which, according to the author, 'every human being knows to be existing within himself' but no one seems able to explain. 'What power', he asks, 'when I am asleep, when my will is entirely inactive, sets this thinking machine going, going as I cannot make it go when my will is active and I am awake?' Collins's perplexity is compounded by the problems of terminology to define the elusive relationship of the 'intellectual faculties, the nerves, and the whole vital principle'. Despite his quandary, he comes close here to hypothesizing what G. H. Lewes, some two decades later, would formulate scientifically, namely the total physiology of the organism as a dynamic interaction of body, mind, and nerves. It might be more accurate to say, on the other hand, that he comes close to anticipating the next raft of insoluble problems.

Social, moral, and psychological notions of disease transmission are as pertinent to Collins's depiction of Basil's sickness as are the physiological hard facts which authenticate its crisis. In mid-century medical circles, the concept of post-traumatic illness was already a well-discussed phenomenon and it was recognized that a shock to the system, whether emotional, spiritual, or caused by physical injury, could give rise to symptoms which, looked at in isolation, might be wrongly attributed to unrelated disease. In clinical terms, Basil's collapse was consistent with the shock of his discovery of the sexual liaison between Margaret and Mannion. The effect upon him is immediate and explicitly physical. 'I could neither move nor breathe', he recalls:

The blood surged and heaved upward to my brain; my heart strained and writhed in anguish; the life within me raged and tore to get free.

[21] *The Leader*, iii. 99 (14 February 1852), 160–1 (p. 161).

Whole years of the direst mental and bodily agony were concentrated in that one moment of helpless, motionless torment. I never lost the consciousness of suffering. I heard the waiter say, under his breath, 'My God! he's dying.' I felt him loosen my cravat—I knew that he dashed cold water over me; dragged me out of the room; and, opening a window on the landing, held me firmly where the night-air blew upon my face. I knew all this; and knew when the paroxysm passed, and nothing remained of it, but a shivering helplessness in every limb. (160–1)

The loss of consciousness which later marks the start of Basil's illness, by contrast, ushers in a variety of darkly imaginative theories linking physical and moral contagion.

In the climate of secrecy, surveillance, and unintelligibility created in this and in later sensational texts, the fear of hidden taint and of invisible agents of disease provides a strong narrative potential as science and popular conjecture contribute, on equal terms, to the task of tracing lines of contamination. Physicians and nerve specialists, familiar with the way in which delirium supervened upon severe organic illness, were always in pursuit of physiological clues to what Prichard had called all the 'phases and varieties of mental alienation'. While there was general recognition that emotional causes could have physical effects, there was still much speculation as to whether sudden, unexpected fevers of the brain might be themselves transmitted through an organic chain. Not surprisingly, the idea that external agents could induce mental pathologies which manifested as organic brain disease carried sinister overtones in a decade as yet ignorant of the precise mechanisms of infection and contagion. According to *The Cyclopaedia of Practical Medicine*, it had been 'incontrovertibly established' that '[t]he human body, not only when affected with disease, but under certain circumstances in a state of health, generates a poison which gives rise to fever'.[22] It was, of course, self-evident that some diseases passed from person to person through physical contact. But prior to the discovery of the micro-organism in the 1880s, modes of transmission were the subject of much inconclusive speculation which was none the less put to the service of many

---

[22] *The Cyclopaedia of Practical Medicine*, ii. p. 192.

a moral or political agenda.[23] We are apt to confuse, warns a writer in the *Westminster Review*, morbid states of panic, fear, and hysterical imitation with those of contagion, 'the contagion having been only real in the same sense as laughter and yawning are contagious'.[24] It is the sense impressions of sight, touch, and smell which convey to the mind the fear, if not the reality, of contagious disease. It is hardly surprising that a writer intent upon amplifying suspense should seize upon the notion of some invisible agent of contamination to manipulate anxiety and the sense of vulnerability. Basil's delirious transfiguration of moral contamination into physical images feeds upon the general uncertainty about these real and imagined agents. Although, at one level, the sequence of events leading up to his delirium dictates the immediate cause, an underlying sense of Basil's own moral, emotional, and social inadequacies persists as the language of delusion, memory, and sexual fantasy implicates the sufferer in a nightmare of his own making.

Sinking into the uncontrollable realms of hallucination, Basil recoils from the horror of bodily contact with the 'two monsters stretching forth their gnarled yellow talons to grasp at us; leaving on their track a green decay, oozing and shining with a sickly light'. As each monster lifts a veil on a 'hideous net-work of twining worms', the dreamer recognizes the taint of corruption on the revealed faces of Margaret and Mannion (173–4). The powerful metaphors of contagion serve, simultaneously, to embody the covert transactions between sexes, classes, and cultures, and to import into Basil's sickness imputations of the moral degeneracy of Margaret and Mannion. Ideas of moral and physical contagion are similarly configured by other writers during the mid-century period. Written only a year after *Basil*, Dickens's *Bleak House* recounts Lady Dedlock's contamination with the deadly diseases emanating from the pauper's graveyard of Tom-All-Alone's while deliberately obscuring the source of moral degeneracy in the entangled skein of inter-class affairs and illegitimacy. Physical and moral contagion are again inextricably

---

[23] For a study of nineteenth-century bacteriology and its incorporation into fiction, see A. Susan Williams, *The Rich Man and the Diseased Poor in Early Victorian Literature* (London: Macmillan, 1987).

[24] 'Electro-biology', *Westminster Review*, 55 (1851), 312–28 (p. 325).

fused in George Eliot's 'The Lifted Veil' when Latimer is overcome with an etherized numbness as the touch of Bertha's hand
on his arm conveys the 'fatal odour' exuding from the portrait of
Lucrezia Borgia.[25] For writers whose work, like that of Collins,
was informed by psychological research, images of disease transmission offered convincing metaphors for the workings of the
human mind in trains of thought, paths, or the association of
ideas. Even as late as 1872, and after association theories had
largely given way to spatial models of consciousness, Sheridan
Le Fanu was causally linking mental afflictions to the inability of
sufferers to break the associative chains which aggravated their
torment and also invoking ideas of contagion to intensify fears
of contracting mental maladies. In his story, 'The Familiar', for
instance, the sufferer, Barton, finds temporary relief from his
terrors only when the 'chain of associations' with which his mind
intensifies his 'obstinate hypochondria' is broken by enforced
social interaction. Earlier, the clergyman listening to Barton's
catalogue of misery warns him not to 'give way to those wild
fancies; [to] resist these impulses of the imagination' when he
senses that 'something disagreeably contagious in the nervous
excitement' of his visitor threatens his own mental health.[26]

   The language with which Collins describes the sounds, movements, and phantasmagoric sensations of Basil's hallucinatory
experience is drawn from a register of symptomatology
compiled from medical and literary encounters with delirium.[27]
Boundaries between clinical and fictional explanations are
collapsed as Collins locates Basil's mental state, both literally
and figuratively, in a liminal landscape where sensations and
impressions, once mediated by rational consciousness, now 'all
acted in the frightful self-concentration of delirium' (169).
Neither fully conscious nor unconscious, the same 'sensations

[25] *Bleak House*, p. 278; 'The Lifted Veil', ed. by Helen Small (Oxford: Oxford
University Press, 1999), p. 19. For a reading of 'contagious disease' in *Bleak House*,
see Graham Benton, ' "And Dying Thus Around Us Every Day": Pathology,
Ontology and the Discourse of the Diseased Body, A Study of Illness and Contagion
in *Bleak House*', *Dickens Quarterly*, 11 (1994), 69–80.
[26] Sheridan Le Fanu, *In A Glass Darkly* (1872), ed. by Robert Tracy (New York:
Oxford University Press, 1993), pp. 71–72, 63.
[27] Jenny Bourne Taylor sources Collins's excursion into the language and images
of hallucinatory experience in Thomas De Quincey's *Confessions of an English
Opium Eater*. See *In the Secret Theatre of Home*, p. 89.

... thoughts ... visions' of conscious, waking life begin to shift and transform their own meanings and the patient's response to them. An idea of an intermediate space within which sensations received from the external world are processed into the thoughts and impressions which shape individual identity is crucial to an understanding of George Eliot's representation of Gwendolen Harleth in *Daniel Deronda*. But the ideas which Eliot was to develop in tandem with the new science of neurology were already taking shape in the 1850s. Writers exploited the phenomenon of altered perception experienced in delirium to present anomalistic or perverse interpretations of the objects of the external world, and of the self in relation to that world.

In recalling his delirium, Basil is at once sufferer and voyeur struggling to make sense of a landscape in which the familiar and unfamiliar merge into one 'hideous phantasmagoria' (169). In the previous chapter I referred to Henry Holland's neurological explanation of distorted perception. When David Brewster reviewed Holland's book, *Chapters on Mental Physiology*, for the *North British Review* in 1854, he raised some interesting questions about the morbid destruction of the channels of communication between the objects of reality and subjective vision. Although he does not use the word 'phantasmagoria', Brewster brings the nightmare visions of individuals who see what is not there and fail to see what is, under the scrutiny of medical diagnosis:

In every case of mental alienation, the ideas which successively rush through the mind are embodied in external phenomena which the senses take cognizance of, as if they were real existences, and which are therefore necessarily the result of reverse impressions made upon the nerves of sensation.[28]

Since, Brewster continues, it is the will which controls and 'directs the organs of sensation to the accurate examination of objects', a healthy and proper balance is seldom the attribute of those 'whose imagination is highly sensitive and morbid' and whose 'mind exercises a very feeble coercive power over the train of its associations'. Similarly, when delirium removes

[28] David Brewster, 'Mental Physiology', *North British Review*, 22 (1854), 179–224 (p. 197).

the controlling will undifferentiated images proliferate in the mind.

In Basil's fevered dreams, old associations are continually made and re-made, enticing the hapless sufferer into thinking that the psychic world will give access to truths hidden from the real one:

> In the clinging heat and fierce seething fever, to which neither waking nor sleeping brought a breath of freshness or a dream of change, I began to act my part over again, in the events that had passed, but in a strangely altered character. Now, instead of placing implicit trust in others, as I had done; instead of failing to discover a significance and a warning in each circumstance as it arose, I was suspicious from the first—suspicious of Margaret, of her father, of her mother, of Mannion, of the very servants in the house. In the hideous phantasmagoria of my own calamity on which I now looked, my position was reversed. Every event of the doomed year of my probation was revived. But the doom itself, the night-scene of horror through which I had passed, had utterly vanished from my memory. This lost recollection, it was the one unending toil of my wandering mind to recover, and I never got it back. None who have not suffered as I suffered then, can imagine with what a burning rage of determination I followed past events in my delirium, one by one, for days and nights together,—followed, to get to the end which I knew was beyond, but which I never could see, not even by glimpses, for a moment at a time. (169–70)

Basil's delirium fails to lift the last veil between the figurative landscape of associations and the perceptive consciousness of ordinary daily life. Instead, his disordered mind takes him back over the events and impressions of the previous year, schizophrenically alternating between the remembrance of a terrible, overwhelming anguish and an entirely new power to perceive his experiences as part of a larger scheme of interconnectedness. The dreamer becomes at once the subject and spectator of his calamity though not its elucidator.

The feeling of traversing back and forth across an indeterminate terrain, seeing and understanding differently, but never knowing for certain, is a feature of delirium common to innumerable fictional and medical accounts. Collins's analogy of the restoration of sight to the blind is powerfully suggestive of the delirious patient's bewilderment when the tantalizing array of 'brilliant colours and ever-varying forms' (168), instead of affording privileged insight, yields nothing which makes sense. In some texts, as here, the remembrance is of an agonizing trial in which the sufferer is faced with an unending series of mental puzzles, each more intractable than the one before. Basil recalls the monumental effort as a 'toiling of obscure thought, ever in the same darkened sphere, ever on the same impenetrable subject, ever failing to reach some distant and visionary result'. Far from being a passive mode, delirium, it seems, demands a great deal of mental toil. Carpenter gives scientific sanction to this observation when he notes that febrile delirium is 'a complete disturbance of the intellectual actions' in which 'the thoughts are not inactive, but rather far more active than in health; they are uncontrolled and wander from one subject to another with extraordinary rapidity; or, taking up one single subject, they twist and turn it in every way and shape, with endless and innumerable repetitions'.[29] Along with the absolute compulsion to try to synthesize the myriad of nameless thoughts into a coherent narrative is the sense of the impenetrability of some intrinsic truth which is always just out of reach. 'It was as if something were imprisoned in my mind', Basil complains, 'and moving always to and fro in it—moving, but never getting free' (169). Dickens's Esther is similarly distressed by the 'great perplexity of endlessly trying to reconcile' the cares of the external world in the inner turmoil of her delirium (543).

In other texts, the inward concentration releases the invalid from the fixed objects that have hindered progress in conscious waking life. It is significant that, in Dickens's *Great Expectations*, it is only in the fever supervening on her burns injuries that Miss Havisham is able to cast off the veil—in her case, literally as well as metaphorically—of intervening years, the veil of blinding hatred and resentment, to restore the time when Estella first came to her. Speaking with the 'terrible vivacity' of a mind sinking into delirium, she finally confronts her error of years and, through the ministrations of Pip, begs for forgiveness. Her tormented mind grasps at the fast-disappearing threads of communication with the outside world, and she mutters 'innumerable times in a low solemn voice':

---

[29] *Principles of Human Physiology*, p. 834.

'What have I done!' And then, 'When she first came, I meant to save her from misery like mine.' And then, 'Take the pencil and write under my name, "I forgive her!" ' She never changed the order of these three sentences, but she sometimes left out a word in one or other of them; never putting in another word, but always leaving a blank and going on to the next word.[30]

In a disconcerting way, these delirious babblings present Miss Havisham in a more human and benevolent light than when guided by the supposed lucidity and coherence of conscious reason. In *Our Mutual Friend*, delirium, once again supervening on bodily trauma, frees the mind from paralysing obsession. Eugene Wrayburn pleads, in the repetitive, distracted utterances of fever, for Bradley Headstone's release from being brought to justice for the near-fatal injuries he inflicted on him. Although primarily driven by his desire to spare his beloved Lizzie Hexam from the taint of association with the manic Headstone, this fever-induced generosity is not directed towards making amends for the errors of the past.[31] Wrayburn's delirious crisis, unlike Miss Havisham's, does not illuminate the need for a recovery or restoration of a previous way of life, so much as the need to accept a new, and hitherto impossible one. In the feverish wanderings of delirium, Miriam Bailin argues, the 'insoluble enigma' that was Eugene Wrayburn's preferred self-designation begins to resolve into a new identity of depleted, dependent, docile decipherability.[32] But in so far as delirium is a site of transformation or adjustment or renewal, the process is one of mental toil rather than passive accommodation. The notion of 'recovery' is more problematic in Dickens than the mere 'survival' of the delirious patient would suggest.

As well as opening the mind to realms beyond normal perception, the phenomenon of delirium reopened the mind to areas of knowledge long since forgotten. Medical writers testify to a far from uncommon occurrence in which those labouring under delirium revive with vivid intensity impressions associated with

---

[30] Charles Dickens, *Great Expectations* (1860–1), ed. by Edgar Rosenberg (New York: W. W. Norton, 1995), p. 300. Subsequent references to this edition will be given in the text.

[31] *Our Mutual Friend*, p. 808.

[32] *The Sickroom in Victorian Fiction: The Art of Being Ill* (Cambridge: Cambridge University Press, 1994), pp. 100–4.

scenes long past and long since erased from the memory. Carpenter is one of many who regaled their readers with the story of a female patient who spoke fluently in Hebrew and Chaldaic, languages of which she was quite ignorant in her fully conscious life.[33] The story is remarkable notwithstanding the fact that it was subsequently explained by her having once been a servant in the home of a clergyman who was accustomed to reading aloud in these languages which, it seems, her memory retained unconsciously. It can be argued, of both Miss Havisham and Pip, that their deliriums bring back into focus circumstances which once prevailed or, more suggestively, that the very loss of a controlling will over the familiar train of their thoughts imparts a new fluency to a fragmented, dislocated self. But the question of the transportability of this new kind of coherence beyond the delirium is a vexed one which turns on the ambiguity of the word 'recovery'. In the case of Pip, we are led to believe that his delirium has effected a transformative function when, on his emergence from the fever, his behaviour and attitude towards Joe have assumed a new humility.[34] Recovery however, seems little more than a consolatory fiction, permitting him to 'fancy' himself 'little Pip again' and 'half-believe' that all the failings of his adult life were the figments of sick dreams (346).

The condition into which the perplexities of a lifetime are temporarily compressed raises questions which search beyond individual suffering to the function of mental life and to its status in relation to the material body. Bringing into closer scrutiny a mental landscape where the images and sensations drawn from waking life are distorted, disordered, and given startling twists of significance and association, delirium alters

---

[33] *Principles of Human Physiology*, p. 808. Carpenter is drawing here on an anecdote which can be traced back to Samuel Taylor Coleridge's *Biographia Literaria* (1817). There are many variations of this story: J. G. Millingen, for instance, substitutes the servant girl for a man struck by the shaft of a cart and taken to St Thomas's hospital with concussion whereupon he begins to speak in a language recognized as Welsh by a Welshman in the same ward. *Mind and Matter, Illustrated by Considerations on Heredity, Insanity, and the Influence of Temperament in the Development of the Passions* (London: H. Hurst, 1847), p. 151.

[34] Miriam Bailin hints at the double sense of 'recovery' when she writes that Pip's 'recovery seems to constitute a recovery of his childhood at Joe's side'. *The Sickroom in Victorian Fiction*, p. 88.

the temporal and spatial perspectives which have secured the invalid in a knowable world. Upon the patient's re-emergence into consciousness, these altered perspectives conduce to altered perceptions of his or her place in the broader context of mental and material life and, in turn, cast doubt on the reliability of all the boundaries by which humankind defines its separateness, autonomy, and control. In *Bleak House*, Esther Summerson's account of her fever underlines the power of hallucinatory experience to derange the chronologies and contingencies which form the stable boundaries of waking life. In Esther's case, the delirium brought on by smallpox has confused the more usual divisions of time in an individual's memory; the divisions between childhood, youth, and adulthood, as well as between significant periods or phases of affecting experience, and replaced them with a single, simple division between the state of health and the state of sickness. She recalls how it seemed that 'there was little or no separation between the various stages of my life which had been really divided by years'. Instead of those categories of years, her life was now split in two by a 'dark lake' with illness on one side, and 'all my experiences, mingled together by the great distance, on the healthy shore' (543). 'I had never known before', she reflects, not only 'how short life really was', but 'into how small a space the mind could put it' (543). The divisions between waking and sleeping are equally blurred. Whatever images are chosen as an analogy for the borderline states, they convey some sense of traversibility. Pip's fluctuation between consciousness of his external circumstance and slipping into the internal recesses of his delirium is figured by Dickens as a passing through something akin to 'the vapour of a lime-kiln' (343). For a period, the mind ranges between levels of consciousness, though with sufficient awareness to describe the experience once the fever has subsided. Esther claims that, even during the most distracting of her hallucinations, she 'knew perfectly at intervals, and I think vaguely at most times' that she was in her bed and could hear herself complaining to Charley, ' "O more of these never-ending stairs, Charley,—more and more—piled up to the sky, I think!" and labouring on again' (544). This double consciousness of suffering and reflection, whereby the patient retains some recollection of what passed during the delirium, destabilizes the notion of unified selfhood as a compatibility of body and mind. Esther's impression, as she narrates her experience of approaching fever, is of a self that exceeds the body's limits, of being 'a little beside myself, though knowing where I was; and I felt confused at times—with a curious sense of fullness, as if I were becoming too large altogether' (496).[35]

Testimonies to an enhanced mode of perception, both of the self and of other existences contiguous to the self, may also expose a terrifying diminution of individual status and purpose in a world which now seems strange. According to Carpenter, one of the features distinguishing delirium from normal dreaming was that the images which appear before the patient's heightened perceptive faculties 'are more vividly conceived-of as having an existence external to the mind, . . . the illusory visual and auditory perceptions having all the force of reality'.[36] In *Great Expectations*, Pip's fever induces hallucinations which profoundly disturb his understanding of the division between himself and the inanimate objects that surround him. He recalls:

That I had a fever and was avoided, that I suffered greatly, that I often lost my reason, that the time seemed interminable, that I confounded impossible existences with my own identity; that I was a brick in the house-wall, and yet entreating to be released from the giddy place where the builders had set me; that I was a steel beam of a vast engine, clashing and whirling over a gulf, and yet that I implored in my own person to have the engine stopped, and my part in it hammered off; that I passed through these phases of disease, I know of my own remembrance, and did in some sort know at the time. (343)

Pip's last remark further confirms the double consciousness of being at once the helpless subject and the aware witness of the dream. Esther recalls a similar experience in which she felt herself to be a bead on a flaming necklace, 'strung together somewhere in great black space' (544), pleading to be released from the 'inexplicable agony' of connection to alien entities in a changed hierarchy. These perceptual aberrations point up once again the ways in which delirium unsettles boundaries, both at the level of individual identity and of broader ontological orthodoxy. In

---

[35] A common experience of delirious patients. *The International Dictionary of Medicine and Biology*, 3 vols. (New York: John Wiley, 1986), i. p. 747.

[36] *Principles of Human Physiology*, p. 835.

Dickens's novels, there are unarguable connections, as Miriam Bailin has shown, between the disorientation and frantic searching experienced in delirium and crises of identity in external, waking life. But how far the knowledge disclosed during dreams assigns a new coherence to a fragmented, uncertain selfhood is more debatable. For Pip and Esther, no less than for Latimer in 'The Lifted Veil', double consciousness is a sign and a symptom of affliction; recalling their extraordinary mental states only renews the agony. As the phenomenon of unconscious brain activity gained general acceptance, the idea that thoughts might be influenced or understanding modified by agencies outside the conscious processes of reasoning was both alarming and intriguing. Even if extraordinary states of consciousness brought no special insight, no privileged knowledge that would be of any subsequent use to the dreamer, they were richly rewarding sources of investigation for the novelist and the medical scientist. These involuntary lapses into a realm of heightened sensation and aberrant perception seemed to hold a key which would, if scientifically examined, elucidate how impulses from the outside world are absorbed into individual consciousness.

Although associationism was superseded by ever more complex theories of mental processes, the notion of unconscious thought was still very much in circulation in the 1870s when *Macmillan's Magazine* published an article by Frances Power Cobbe entitled 'Unconcious Cerebration: A Psychological Study'.[37] As the century advanced, ideas about the mysterious boundaries between waking and sleeping, between health and disease, between external reality and private perception, and between conscious volition and unconscious reaction, became increasingly influenced by the biological realism that was integral to evolutionary theory. The discussion which follows takes account of this development and particularly of the physiological implications for mental life which many of George Eliot's scientific contemporaries were striving to establish.[38]

[37] 'Unconscious Cerebration: A Psychological Study', *Macmillan's Magazine*, 23 (1870), 24–37.
[38] For a detailed analysis of the developments in psychology from associationism to psychophysiology, see Robert M. Young, *Mind, Brain and Adaptation in the Nineteenth Century: Cerebral Localization and Its Biological Context from Gall to Ferrier* (Oxford: Clarendon Press, 1970).

THE 'MYSTIC BOUNDARY' BETWEEN BODY AND MIND:
GEORGE ELIOT AND G. H. LEWES

Unlike Dickens's or Collins's investigations into the mysteries of consciousness, Eliot's representation of Gwendolen Harleth in *Daniel Deronda* is not a first-person narrative. Nor does it feature delirium. But as an exploration of the processes by which the objective facts of the external world are assimilated into consciousness, Eliot's last novel is a pioneering literary endeavour incorporating many of the ideas and questions at the forefront of debate in scientific circles and conducting, in the study of Gwendolen, the author's most searching enquiry into the nature of the relationship between body and mind. One of the consequences of her work with Lewes, her close friendships with eminent scientists, doctors and scholars, as well as her curiosity about the more controversial branches of medical science, was an informed engagement with the way in which new research in physiology and psychology impacted upon broader conceptualizations of matter and mind.[39] Inspired by the idea of a physiology of consciousness and, at the same time, maintaining a sceptical resistance to the material dictates of scientific positivism, Eliot carries the spatial analogies, so profitably explored by Collins, into the age of neurological specialism.

As nerve specialists sought to replace what seemed to them largely conjectural causal links between physical and mental states with a more definitive nervous anatomy, the network of the nerves came to be recognized as the mechanism which translated invisible impulses into action, behaviour, and even thought. The work of the neurologist and alienist physician Henry Maudsley embodies in every sense the shift away from speculative notions of 'nerve force' as some immaterial essence

---

[39] The vast collection of mainly scientific works owned by Eliot and Lewes are held in The George Eliot–George Henry Lewes Library in Dr Williams's Library, London. Among them are the works of Henry Maudsley, James Sully, Alexander Bain, Herbert Spencer, Henry Holland, Robert Brudenell Carter, James Paget, and many others indicative of Eliot's and Lewes's lifelong interest in medical science. The collection is catalogued by William Baker, *The George Eliot–George Henry Lewes Library: An Annotated Catalogue of Their Books at Dr. Williams' Library, London* (New York: Garland Publishing, 1977).

of exchange. What he and other devotees of somaticism sought to correct in the earlier explanations of brain and nerve function are evidenced in Brewster's summary of Henry Holland's reflections on cerebral physiology:

> In every treatise on intellectual phenomena, our organs of sensation are supposed to have fulfilled their highest purpose when they have conveyed to the brain the impressions which they receive from external objects. The ideas which thus enter the storehouse of the mind are reproduced in the acts of conception, memory, and imagination; but by what means they are reproduced, through what channel they are presented to us, and in what position and direction they appear in absolute space, are questions the solution of which has not been attempted. According to the views which we have been led to form, the organs of sense are the channels by which these ideas are reproduced; . . . The membranes of sensation, therefore, are the mystic boundary between the two worlds of matter and mind. They receive the impressions of external nature, and convey them to the mind, and, by a similar process they take back and give an external existence to those ideas which the mind desires to be reproduced for intellectual and social purposes.[40]

Maudsley's contribution to the understanding of the problematic relationship of body and mind lies in a positivism which was instrumental in producing increasingly biologistic theories of human behaviour during the second half of the century. No one was more convinced than he of the physicality of mind. We are in error, he writes, in supposing our impressions, emotions, memory, and volition to be faculties of some 'intangible entity or incorporeal essence which science inherited from theology'. Rather, they are organic processes fundamentally indistinguishable from 'the lower nerve centres' which organize our physical life.[41]

Physiologists and psychologists, finding themselves with the task of mapping common territory, coined seemingly ambiguous terminologies such as 'mental physiology' or 'the physical basis of mind' to try to encapsulate properties and principles which they readily acknowledged but were unable to define.[42]

---

[40] 'Mental Physiology', p. 191.
[41] *Body and Mind: An Enquiry Into Their Connection and Mutual Influence, Specially in Reference to Mental Disorders*, being the Gulstonian Lectures for 1870 (London: Macmillan, 1870), pp. 2, 18–19.
[42] Referring to his 1852 work, *Chapters on Mental Physiology*, Henry Holland

In 1855, Henry Holland had presented George Henry Lewes with his *Medical Notes and Reflections*, the concluding remarks of which anticipate the advantage to the physiologists in the boundary dispute:

But between these purely mental inquiries, and those which regard the physical nature of man, there lies an *interspace*; destined ever to continue such; yet greatly narrowed, we may affirm, by the remarkable discoveries regarding the functions of the nervous system, and their relation to mental as well as physical phenomena, which of late years have given a new character to physiology. While recognising still a line and limit, impassable by human reason or research, we have approached nearer to it on this side, and are justified in believing that the same investigation, further pursued, will bring us yet closer to the boundary.[43]

Twenty-two years later, Lewes was confident that his experiments in neurophysiology meant that the 'interspace' was now much better understood. In previous times, he writes:

The logical distinction between Matter and Mind was accepted as an essential distinction, i.e., representing distinct reals. There was on the one side a group of phenomena, Matter and Force; on the other side an unallied group, Feeling and Thought: between them an impassable gulf. How the two were brought into relation, each acting on the other, was dismissed as an 'insoluble mystery'—or relegated to Metaphysics for such minds as chose to puzzle over questions not amenable to experiment.[44]

In a sense, Lewes merely exchanges one imponderable for another when his scientific researches lead him to reject both exclusively biological and exclusively mentalist theories of agency in human behaviour. The study of psychology as an independent science which regarded 'mind' as a purely abstract concept he considers misguided and meaningless. Equally, he is guarded about the extreme somaticist convictions of positivist

explains that he used 'the term to express more especially the reciprocal action and relations of mental and bodily phenomena, as they exist in, and make up the totality of, human life', *Medical Notes and Reflections*, p. 614. *The Physical Basis of Mind* is the title Lewes gave to the second series in his *Problems of Life and Mind* in 1877.

43 *Medical Notes and Reflections*, p. 614, emphasis in original.
44 *The Physical Basis of Mind* (London: Trübner, 1877), p. 309.

physicians such as Maudsley.[45] He became more convinced of the interdependence of body and mind with the nervous system forming the bridge across that once 'impassable' gulf. His preferred model was one of a mediating interspace of nervous function, within which a nerve is 'essentially an exciter of change', an agent of impulse whose activation affects the entire organism.[46] Lewes eventually discarded the metaphor of bridge and gulf altogether and contended that material and mental life were merely the convex and concave aspects of one phenomenon, a position, as Richard Menke points out, 'now known as dual-aspect monism'.[47] In 1876, Lewes contributed an article to the *Fortnightly Review* in which he declared himself to be a confirmed organicist in the debates about the nature of mental life, much to the disapproval of the associational psychologist G. C. Robertson, who continued, none the less, to publish Lewes's work in progress for *The Physical Basis of Mind* in the professional journal *Mind*, of which he was editor.[48] Neither Lewes nor Eliot, though, conceived of physiological psychology as in any sense reductively somatic. On the contrary, physiology was, by definition, the science of the living relationship of body and mind within an environment and was not, therefore, simply reducible to a set of material structures.[49]

A model of an inner network of nerves governing the mind's consciousness of sentient facts is translated by Eliot into literary narrative in the form of a problematic interspace where objective reality and subjective response come together to produce

[45] See Lewes, *The Foundations of a Creed*, 2 vols. (London: Trübner, 1874–5), i. pp. 125–7.

[46] *The Physical Basis of Mind*, p. 176. Despite this title, Lewes, no less than Maudsley, had difficulty in defining abstract phenomena such as 'spirituality' or 'will' in physical terms (that is, as neural acts).

[47] 'Fiction as Vivisection: G. H. Lewes and George Eliot', *ELH*, 67/2 (2000), p. 623.

[48] 'Spiritualism and Materialism', *Fortnightly Review*, o.s. 25 (April, 1876), 479–93 and (May, 1876), 707–19. See Rosemary Ashton, *G. H. Lewes: A Life* (Oxford: Clarendon Press, 1991), pp. 271–2.

[49] In her discussion of 'Mind and Body in *Middlemarch*', Karen Chase sets Eliot's representation of Lydgate's desire to probe the inner mysteries of the mind through better understanding of the body into the contemporary context of scientific positivism, and writes: 'Neither Comte nor Lewes could have put the physiological thesis more concisely'. *Eros and Psyche: The Representation of Personality in Charlotte Brontë, Charles Dickens, and George Eliot* (London: Methuen, 1984), p. 150.

conflicting versions of perspective and interpretation. The vague and analogous descriptions of the nature of the nervous mechanism admit sufficient ambiguity to be transported into fiction in a usefully enigmatic form which, in turn, provides a rationale for Eliot's interrogative methodology in *Daniel Deronda*. Gwendolen's predicament in particular, and the human predicament in general, are cast in the form of neurological mysteries in which the nerves hold the key to the explanation of psychological states. For instance, the measure of Gwendolen's powerlessness to withstand and defy Grandcourt's will is set in direct proportion to the poor quality of her nerves when it is observed that: 'She longed to do it. But she might as well have tried to defy the texture of her nerves and the palpitation of her heart' (447).[50] And, on the larger scale of human stimulus and response, the neurologists' attempts to answer metaphysical perplexities with neurological facts can be heard echoing through such claims as that which troubles the narrator on the matter of Lush's professed insight into the character and motivation of his patron, Grandcourt. Lush, Grandcourt's lackey, claimed to know his master with an inside knowledge that comes after years of close study in a relationship akin to that of the dissector and his specimen.[51] Questioning Lush's 'general certainties' about Grandcourt's inner psychological make-up, the narrator asks, 'Of what use, however, is a general certainty that an insect will not walk with his head hindmost, when what you need to know is the play of inward stimulus that sends him hither and thither in a network of possible paths?' (282). Eliot's exploration of Gwendolen's nervous organization develops the metaphor of the network into more complex concepts. Here, the nerves are directly allied to consciousness. Very much in line with contemporary neurological theory, Eliot understood the nerves to be the operating mechanism converting sense experience into healthy or diseased consciousness.

In *Daniel Deronda*, physiological psychology is replicated in the various dichotomies of inner and outer experience, as

[50] George Eliot, *Daniel Deronda* (1876), ed. by Terence Cave (Harmondsworth: Penguin, 1995). Subsequent references to this edition will be given in the text.

[51] For a persuasive reading equating Eliot's close scrutiny of her characters with the experimental techniques of the vivisectionist, see Richard Menke, 'Fiction as Vivisection: G. H. Lewes and George Eliot'.

Gwendolen's 'inner life' of the nerves, to use Lewes's words, is explored in relation to the influences of the social environment.[52] For many years, the question of agency with regard to the internal and external stimuli which shape individual perception was one which had intrigued Eliot. Her fascination with spiritualist matters kept alive in her mind the problem of interpreting psychic experience within an authoritative frame of scientific reference. To her correspondent and friend Harriet Beecher Stowe, Eliot had written on 24 June 1872:

Perhaps I am inclined, under the influence of the facts, physiological and psychological, which have been gathered of late years, to give larger place to the interpretation of vision-seeing as *subjective* than the Professor would approve. It seems difficult to limit—at least to limit with any precision—the possibility of confounding sense by impressions, derived from inward conditions, with those which are directly dependent on external stimulus. In fact, the division between within and without in this sense seems to become every year a more subtle and bewildering problem.[53]

That expressed bewilderment grew as developments in medical science worked towards definitions of inner psychological states increasingly in terms of the quality of neurological processes.

Eliot's portrayal of Gwendolen's 'peculiar sensitiveness' to the events of the physical world is informed by the positivist physiologists' explanations of behaviour and response. But at the same time, these explanations are shown to be insufficient in their attempts to encompass all mental life within realist principles. Throughout, Eliot's study of psychological breakdown ranges across the 'mystic boundary', positing and challenging alike the theories of superstition and of science. The lameness of the one is matched only by the deficiency of the other. Thus, to the unscientific mind, Gwendolen's nature is easily explained:

To her mamma and others her fits of timidity or terror were sufficiently accounted for by her 'sensitiveness' or the 'excitability of her nature;' but these explanatory phrases required conciliation with much that seemed to be blank indifference or rare self-mastery. Heat is a

[52] *Problems of Life and Mind*, 3rd series, vol. 2, p. 139.
[53] *The George Eliot Letters*, v. p. 280, emphasis in original. Eliot's reference to the professor is to Calvin E. Stowe, an eminent biblical scholar and Harriet Beecher Stowe's husband.

great agent and a useful word, but considered as a means of explaining the universe it requires an extensive knowledge of differences; and as a means of explaining character 'sensitiveness' is in much the same predicament. (64)

But science has its limitations, too, when it comes to accounting for human actions and emotions. Whilst it is acknowledged by the narrator that Gwendolen's feelings of personal tragedy when the family fortune is lost and she faces the choice of becoming a governess or selling her jewellery has more to do with her general sense of hopelessness about her influence in the world than with recent events, her immediate reactions are prompted by the 'vague and yet mastering' forces of superstition. With its power to compel individuals to action against all reason, superstition is an agent which must be reckoned 'in spite of theory and science' (276–7).

The value of different forms of knowledge and the quality of the processes by which the facts and events of the outside world are internalized by Gwendolen are questions which remain implicit in Eliot's examination of the power of unconscious forces to determine human behaviour. They form the basis of thematic conflict between what Lewes had termed the 'objective aspect of sentient facts' and the subjective experience of those same facts.[54] It is within what Athena Vrettos has called 'the uncharted spaces between physical reality and psychological interpretations of that reality' that Eliot constructs Gwendolen's neurosis.[55] Incongruity and conflict between inside and outside, between psychological autonomy and hereditary determinism, between moral self-management and haunting dreads, and between egoism and social duty, are the endlessly generating enigmas of the novel and the exacerbating criteria of nervous disease. They are played out in that 'great deal of unmapped country within us which would have to be taken into account in an explanation of our gusts and storms' (277).

Vrettos's use of the word 'neurosis' is slightly more specific than I wish to be. Whilst it is true that Gwendolen is patholog-

---

[54] *The Study of Psychology* (London: Trübner, 1879), p. 14. Lewes's research for this book was under way in 1876. It was, of course, published posthumously.
[55] Athena Vrettos, *Somatic Fictions: Imagining Illness in Victorian Culture* (Stanford: Stanford University Press, 1995), p. 61.

ically self-obsessed and her suffering is real enough, my reading is concerned to examine the extent to which Eliot, like Lewes, understood the emotional and psychological life as directly responsive to, and inseparable from, physiology and environment. As the agents of exchange between the various aspects of individual experience—psychological, physiological, and social—the nerves are, in a very important sense, an 'unmapped country'. In Gwendolen, Eliot examines the very processes which eluded much scientific theorizing. Most medical writers were puzzled as to the dynamic relation of impulse and will in nervous organization, and, in the absence of terminologies for such concepts, found themselves falling back onto the figurative language of literature.[56] Even Maudsley's disapproval of what he regards as the meaningless abstractions of metaphysics does not insure him against using language more prevalent in sensation fiction. His declaration 'that everything which is displayed outwardly is contained secretly in the innermost', though offered as a straightforward statement of neurological fact, is imbued with a sense of mystique.[57] Indeed, the representation of Gwendolen's nervous organization by means of a third-person interrogative, and implicitly interpretative, narration suggests a more complex, and perhaps ultimately imperceptible, dynamic than that which science is able to reveal. It is tempting to imagine that the question posed in the opening sentence of the novel—'what was the secret of form or expression which gave the dynamic quality to her glance?'—is one which Maudsley might have felt himself qualified to answer. For Richard Menke, it is this interrogative opening which immediately alerts us to Eliot's concerns with 'measuring', 'reckoning', and 'assessing' the female consciousness, and thus sets the novel firmly within the vivisectionist controversies in which Lewes was involved both implicitly, through his experimental work,

---

[56] 'Although some attempts were made to encapsulate the will within a vaguely somatic description, such as "neural act" ', writes Janet Oppenheim, it refused to fit into any established category of nervous organization. Maudsley, she notes, 'notoriously impatient with what he considered an "irrational dualism" . . . nonetheless himself published a book entitled *Body and Will* in 1883. Despite his concerted efforts throughout the volume, he was unable to make the will coterminous with a cluster of nervous centers in the brain'. *'Shattered Nerves': Doctors, Patients, and Depression in Victorian England* (New York: Oxford University Press, 1991), p. 43.

[57] *Body and Mind*, p. 24.

and directly, through his testifying before a Royal Commission.[58] Close scrutiny of Gwendolen's inner life is not enough, in itself, any more than was Lydgate's microscopic scrutiny of the molecular structure of tissues in *Middlemarch*, to reveal the functioning of the whole organism. Eliot is more concerned to understand that which cannot be seen—but which exerts a powerful determining influence over human behaviour—on the basis of what is seen. Crucially, then, when Lewes describes the neural activity of the inner life as 'the silent growth of *tendencies*', his memorable phrase encapsulates both the scientist's vision of internal processes of transformation operating beyond the control of the will, and the less scientifically assured sense of 'vague and yet mastering' workings of impulse which charged the psychological narratives of Eliot's fictions.[59]

Notions of tendency are central to Eliot's exposition of Gwendolen's fluctuating states of mind. Despite the psychological overtones which the term 'tendency' imparts, it hints also at a physiological powerlessness in the submission to overmastering organic forces.[60] In this second sense, 'tendency' is powerfully suggestive of constitutional predisposition and it is no coincidence that physiologists researching disease aetiology took encouragement from evolutionary biology and turned their attention from the body as a single entity, pressed upon by circumstance and environment, to more distant atavistic sources. Eliot's representation of nervousness draws upon the model of a neurological network of mental pathology but highlights the contradictions, ambiguities, and indeterminacies which continued to unsettle purely somatic designations of health and disease. By delineating a form of emotional and psychological breakdown that is always potential rather than fully realized, Eliot locates Gwendolen's inner experience within contemporary controversies over the organic reality of neurotic disorders. Residual elements of the kind of sexual stereotyping which led doctors to diagnose cases of female hysteria continue

[58] 'Fiction as Vivisection: G. H. Lewes and George Eliot', p. 637.

[59] *Problems of Life and Mind*, 3rd series, vol. 2, p. 24, emphasis in original.

[60] Tend, from Latin *tendere*, carries both connotations: a physical movement in some direction or towards some point, and a psychological inclination or disposition. *OED*.

to charge Eliot's representation of, for instance, Gwendolen's wilfulness, desire for mastery and distaste for marriage, her outbursts of violent passion, and the morbid self-obsession which medicine traditionally assigned, along with mystic and premonitory powers, to that archetypal female neurosis. But Eliot provides an intricate analysis of physiological psychology which probes far beyond these simple symptomatologies and is closely in line with Lewes's science. Gwendolen's vacillations, unpredictability, incongruity between outward appearance and inner turmoil present a more complex picture of the physiological interconnectedness of body and mind and, consequently, more difficult problems of interpretation and therapeutics. This is the study of a woman whose actions and reactions were not in themselves pathological, but always in the process of becoming so. The question of the nature and source of her pain is a hermeneutic conundrum which, just like that of whether she was 'beautiful or not beautiful' (7), pressingly demands to be answered by all observers and commentators. Eliot's contention is that it remains unanswerable in absolute terms, and instead always subject to multiple perspectives.

'CONTRARY TENDENCIES': PHYSIOLOGICAL PSYCHOLOGY IN *DANIEL DERONDA*

Gwendolen's suffering is configured in crises of alienation and detachment from the continuities and contingencies by which the external world is understood. With characteristic anxiety, her sense of self is fragmented between being able to perceive herself only 'in that reflected way' (39) from knowing that one is admired, and an imperceptible centre harbouring a 'soul burning with a sense of what the universe is not' (53). Her predicament lies in the very ambiguity of the qualities by which she is defined, so that her desired public image of exceptionality of 'nerve' is constantly undermined by her liability to 'nervousness'. From the start, Gwendolen's difference is registered in the texture of her nerves. Set apart both from other women, and, as Barbara Hardy notes, from previous Eliot heroines, by her 'nervous equipment', Gwendolen is characterized by her 'peculiar sensitiveness' (25) or 'that liability of hers to fits of spiritual dread' (63).[61] These dubious properties, on the other hand, are regarded by Gwendolen as attributes, indeed as 'a mark of her general superiority' (25). Incongruities between appearance and her own feelings hint at the play of 'contrary tendencies' which confuse observers and Gwendolen alike. While 'she had the charm, and those who feared her were also fond of her; the fear and fondness' were mingled in 'what may be called the iridescence of her character' (42). Elaborating on the opinion of the governess, Miss Merry, the narrator remarks that, whilst other people might be willing to 'have their lives blown hither and thither like empty ships in which no will was present: it was not to be so with her'. Contrarily, this 'delicate-limbed sylph of twenty', for all her 'feminine furniture', is a woman who 'meant to lead', to 'conquer circumstances by her exceptional cleverness' (39). Obsessed with mastery, she disdains the common lot of her sex, preferring to be seen excelling at more active pursuits. Archery and hunting on a spirited mount, together with the recklessness of gambling, are acts of rebellion against domesticity and invisibility which, as Bonnie Zimmerman remarks, 'excite her even as they unsex and almost declass her'.[62] If this is true, they are the very same acts long-presumed by medical theoreticians to precipitate female nervous ills. The thorny issue of the female will establishes itself in the text as qualitatively different from the male will—traditionally construed as the steadfastness of purpose concomitant with more stable and healthy nerves. Lacking the necessary nervous equipment for rational conduct, the female will, thought to be governed solely by feeling and impulse, was considered to require reining in. Gwendolen's fear of what she might do, given free rein to her passions and imaginings, is persistently present in the repeated images of the tightly reined horse. While her equestrian skill marks her out as something exceptional, the image of the horse and rider is a familiar one in

---

[61] See Barbara Hardy's Introduction to *Daniel Deronda* (Penguin, 1967), p. 27.

[62] Bonnie Zimmerman, 'Gwendolen Harleth and "The Girl of the Period" ', in Anne Smith (ed.), *George Eliot: Centenary Essays and an Unpublished Fragment* (London: Vision Press, 1980), pp. 196–217 (p. 209). The first of a series of articles entitled 'The Girl of the Period' had appeared in the *Saturday Review* in 1868. Written by the staunchly antifeminist Eliza Lynn Linton, the articles painted a derogatory picture of the emerging 'New Woman'.

contemporary writings on volition and bodily reflexes. It was an image used by Carpenter in *Principles of Mental Physiology* (1874), a revised version of the book to which I have earlier referred, in order to explain the relationship between the involuntary actions of the nerves and the controlling power or absence of the will.[63] Used here by Eliot, it immediately announces the danger of assuming a continuity between outward display and inward vitality. As the fragility of Gwendolen's self-esteem is exposed through the thin veneer of the sparkling social exterior, the texture of her nerves is increasingly pathologized.

The sense of the impenetrability of nervous disease, due to the bewildering catalogue of signs ranged at the borderline between outward behaviour and inner impulse, is communicated in Gwendolen's 'iridescence', a quality which makes manifest the play of seeming contradictions and raises again the concept of double consciousness. Eliot's conceptualization of the interplay of forces corresponds with Lewes's own experiments demonstrating that the nervous organism was affected equally by conscious interactions with the environment and unconscious impulses. Along with other physiologists, he hypothesized the existence of double, or even multiple, levels of impulse and motivation. If, as he believed, every sensation, every impression, modifies the neural activity in the brain, then reflexes, both physical and psychological, might be explained as memorized reactions to signals acquired over time, or, as Lewes prefers, reactivations of the 'residue of past experiences'. Sensorial traces in the memory, of which the individual is entirely unconscious, he suggests, 'count among the motors of the inner life' which operate outside the controlling influence of the will. Lewes extends this concept to allow him to argue that 'unconsciousness' is a state of mind which, logically, should be included 'within the sphere of sentience'.[64] That the individual is motivated at some level by unconscious impulses was not

[63] See Sally Shuttleworth, *George Eliot and Nineteenth-Century Science: The Make-Believe of a Beginning* (Cambridge: Cambridge University Press, 1984), p. 188.
[64] G. H. Lewes, *Problems of Life and Mind*, 3rd series, vol. 2, pp. 270, 97, and 153. See also Alexander Bain, *Mind and Body: The Theories of Their Relation* (London: Henry S. King, 1873).

new, of course, as the discussion of 'unconscious cerebration' earlier in this chapter makes clear. But that it was the subject of intense interest and speculation is perhaps not surprising since the idea of impulse as a residual trace seemed more probable in the light of contemporary theories of hereditary determinism. Lewes's axiom of the 'silent growth of tendencies', designating those impulses which had the power of imperceptibly transforming and determining, but which themselves remained ungovernable, unamenable to the will, had a fascinating, if sinister, plausibility. It is not difficult to see the close similarity of these enquiries into the respective influence of immediate and more distant 'motors of the inner life' and Eliot's portrayal of an individual whose psychological well-being is increasingly eroded by ungovernable impulses of hereditary transmission.

These ideas gained currency, especially after 1871, when Darwinian theory of descent and sexual selection seemed to ratify the alleged connection between nervous constitution and the incapacity of the female will.[65] Encouraged by the prospect of tracing psychological weaknesses back to biological sources, medical men began to pursue the family history of patients in order to chart the course of nervous disease. According to the evolutionary physicians, there was no escape from the morbid reciprocity of physiological and psychological inheritance which, it was claimed, severely restricted a woman's capability of self-determination. Such doctrines were to dominate the cognitive and perceptual revisions of the nervous body in the last quarter of the century. They reinforced a suspicion (much elaborated in popular fiction) that functional disorder may be the manifestation not simply of a nervous susceptibility inherent in the individual, but of a neurotic tendency which has its origins much further back in ancestral weaknesses. Above all, they revived old myths and prejudices about sexual difference and gender so that the belief in masculine endowment with physical prowess, mental acuity, and logical analysis, and feminine domination of intellect by intuition and feeling seemed to be strengthened by the laws of natural selection. Science had given 'fresh vigour' to half-formulated notions of continuity and

---

[65] Charles Darwin, *The Descent of Man, and Selection in Relation to Sex* (1871), 2nd edn. (London: John Murray, 1883).

kinship, notes Eliot's narrator. This was a time when 'the soul of man was waking to pulses which had for centuries been beating in him unheard' and when girls such as Gwendolen Harleth are the 'delicate vessels' destined by nature to bear 'onward through the ages the treasure of human affections' (124). Eliot's study of diseased consciousness explores the implications for the individual sufferer of this new dimension in nervous pathology. While recapitulating points made by Gillian Beer in her influential study of evolutionary narrative in nineteenth-century fiction, my interpretation emphasizes different aspects of a burden of inheritance which Eliot articulates through contemporary neurological theories of the physiology of consciousness.[66]

In her discussion of *Daniel Deronda*, Beer analyses Gwendolen's nervous dreads in the context of the oppressive determinism which Darwinian theory now cast upon such matters as physiological inheritance, sexual selection, and social integration.[67] Viewed from a medical perspective, evolutionary theory prioritized the linear and temporal dimension of disease over the spatial. In other words, the attention of diagnosticians turned to the criteria of heredity with more hope of unlocking the secrets of nervous debility than the isolated interpretation of immediate symptoms seemed to afford. On a conceptual level, this change is bound up with contemporary theories of organicism, of viewing the body not as a separate entity but as necessarily involved in the totality of social and biological history. The enthusiasm of evolutionary physicians for the pursuit of atavistic explanations of debility encouraged a narrative of neurosis which could be traced along a continuous development and was, in that respect, dynamically different from one which regarded nervous breakdown as an isolated aberration. Importantly, the linear dimension of disease definition was consistent with theories about the relativity of pathology to physiology, theories which Eliot encountered largely through the writings of Claude Bernard. The significance of these ideas

---

[66] Gillian Beer, *Darwin's Plots: Evolutionary Narrative in Darwin, George Eliot and Nineteenth-Century Fiction* (London: Ark Paperbacks, 1985. First published 1983).

[67] Beer writes: 'In *Daniel Deronda* descent and extension are the ordering principles—and simultaneously its unsolvable problems'. *Darwin's Plots*, p. 182.

will become more apparent, but the point to be made here is that debate turned on the question of whether morbid pathology existed as an essentially different condition, the 'opposite' of healthy physiology, or, alternatively, as a continuum, that is to say, quantitatively but not qualitatively different from the normal. Eliot's delineation of Gwendolen's 'difference' shows an awareness of the conceptual possibilities advanced in this debate whereby, according to Bernard and Lewes, differences of principle are negotiated into a system of perspective. Whilst it is the texture of Gwendolen's nerves that becomes the index against which the indeterminate relationship between health and disease is explored, it is in their operation that the breakdown between physiology or, as Lewes put it, the 'objective aspect of sentient facts' and psychological response or '[subjective] states of Feeling' takes place.[68]

Above all, it is Gwendolen's overwhelming dreads which signal her potential for nervous disease. Eliot's theme of dreads is represented as a pathological perversion of the Darwinian explanation of fear. Fear, being a primitive emotion, serves no purpose in the race for survival in the developed world of the nineteenth century. Indeed, Gwendolen's 'large discourse of imaginative fears' (423) puts her at a disadvantage, as Beer notes, in her dealings with Grandcourt's will and with the management of her own choices.[69] Gwendolen's dread of Grandcourt serves no purpose other than to exacerbate her own morbid impressions and is indicative of the degeneration of the primitive mechanism by which disabling terror is transmuted into the 'constructive vindictiveness' (673) deemed necessary for survival. Thus, when Deronda advises: 'Turn your fear into a safeguard. Keep your dread fixed on the idea of increasing your remorse' (674), Gwendolen is quite unable to liberate her private malevolent thoughts from a narrative of vengeance in which the catalogue of her 'past wrong-doing' is deemed to be instrumental in precipitating events. Deronda's counsel is misconstrued so that, far from working therapeutically, it merely serves to augment her guilt. With the characteristic interiority of the nervous temperament, Gwendolen is overtaken by

[68] G. H. Lewes, *The Study of Psychology*, p. 14.
[69] *Darwin's Plots*, p. 228.

an inappropriate and disproportionate response to the objects, ideas, and probabilities outside the self. Her dread is an object-less, self-generating form of fear which dissipates self-determi-nation into 'sick motivelessness' (274), a symptom which Henry Maudsley, among many others, associated with the condition known as 'morbid egoism'. Sufferers labouring under this disor-der are liable to distort the objects, ideas, and events of the world outside the self into a false perception of the relationship of those objective facts to the self. When Eliot's narrator remarks on passions which have been allowed to germinate like fertile seeds to 'a predominance which determines all currents towards itself' (673), the analysis is one that is reiterated time and again by commentators on all forms of morbid introspec-tion ranging from 'mild egoism' to 'insane neurosis'.

Maudsley identified a correlation between patients he diag-nosed as 'egotistic beings' and incipient insanity. Those individ-uals who are 'entrenched within their morbid self-feeling', he claimed, are destined by nature to become sick.[70] 'The associa-tion of morbid introspection, exaggerated self-consciousness, and "unnatural egoism" with mental disorder', Michael Clark notes, 'was thus fundamental, even causal' and not 'merely symptomatic or accidental'.[71] For the majority of Victorian medical psychologists, the real threat to healthy functioning lay in the exercise of a vivid imagination without the due moderat-ing influence of the will, so that a point is ultimately reached when rational judgement of external phenomena is superseded by irrational fear. A psychiatric model which distinguished between 'object-consciousness' as the defining feature of health and 'subject-consciousness' as that of morbidity and degenera-tion was almost unanimously supported. It is worth recalling at this point the explanation of the altered perspectives encountered during states of delirium as being due to the inward turning of the mind away from consciousness of external objects and events. The principle of relating interiority to disease and exteri-ority to health is one which underlies Eliot's differentiation of

[70] Henry Maudsley, *Body and Mind*, pp. 64–5.
[71] Michael Clark, ' "Morbid Introspection": Unsoundness of Mind, and British Psychological Medicine, *c.*1830–*c.*1900', in *The Anatomy of Madness: Essays in the History of Psychiatry*, iii. pp. 71–101 (p. 75).

Gwendolen's psychological organization from that of Deronda, or of Mirah or Mordecai.[72]

Although Eliot uses the words 'fear' and 'dread' interchangeably, she distinguishes quite clearly between rational and objectless forms. Gwendolen's sexual, social, and cultural difference is registered in the disabling effects of her dread. As with Deronda, dread is associated with a rootlessness that is continually signalled in an uncertain genealogy. 'It was', we are told, 'the habit of his mind to connect dread with unknown parentage' (207). But where Deronda's psychic history evolves from unknown origins towards integration into a community, Gwendolen's 'discourse of imaginative fears' propels her into psychic disunity. The 'griefs of inheritance' which weigh within Deronda are directed outside the self through rational consideration and not through impulse. His anxiety on Mirah's behalf is neither vague nor indeterminate, but has fixed reference points in origin and discovery. Similarly, Mirah's memories of how, as a child, she 'made a life in my own thoughts quite different from everything about me' (213) express not so much a form of mental alienation as a profound sense of dissolution into the illimitable matrix of Jewish kinship and commerce. But Gwendolen's dreads are of quite another order, and more compatible with the kind of pathological misinterpretation of impressions documented in medical textbooks.

Governed more by impulse than rational interpretation, Gwendolen's terror of being 'alone in the night' (55) and of any 'rapid change in the light' (63) attests to the ominous non-specificity of her dread. Untroubled by fear 'in action and companionship' (71), her sickness is generated in the self-referencing spaces of morbid introspection, causing her to admit to Deronda to being 'frightened at myself' (452), or of what she might become. When the imagination finds no outlet in creativity, it exercises itself by searching for meaning and significance where there are none, with the result that the healthy assimilation of objective reality into subjective perception turns into

---

[72] The terms 'object-consciousness' and 'subject-consciousness' were coined by William Bevan Lewis in *A Textbook of Mental Diseases* (London: Charles Griffin, 1889), but these, and related sets of associations and contrasts such as 'introversion/extroversion', 'egoism/altruism', were repeatedly invoked (before Lewis) to construct a model of health and disease.

pathogenic transformation. It is just such a breakdown in the mind's capacity for distinguishing between the real and imaginary, the significant and the inconsequential, that is indicated in Gwendolen, of whom it is observed that 'all this yeasty mingling of dimly understood facts with vague but deep impressions, and with images half real, half fantastic' (354) vied within her consciousness for priority. Hierarchies collapse and time is compressed as the impressions generated in moments of self-absorption push into 'hazy perspective' the events and significances of external reality. Since the early decades of the century, physicians had been warning of the perils of imagination unchecked by rational judgement. Where Carpenter had identified the characteristics which distinguished delirium from normal dreaming, Eliot's friend James Sully attempted to establish a physiological basis within the individual for the disturbing perceptual aberrations of the distracted mind. 'All the phenomena of mysterious presentiments, supernatural warnings, and vague forebodings', he wrote in 1874, may be traced back, not to a past reality, but to a 'subjective origin'.[73] On the day of Gwendolen's marriage to Grandcourt, internal impressions take on a reality which breaks through the veneer of Gwendolen's outer brilliance and disturbs the complacency with which she had hitherto defined herself as an object of admiration. Nervous dreads have transformed Gwendolen's youthful egoism into neurotic self-absorption, which effectively dislocates her from the progressive narratives of healthy self-fulfilment and aligns her instead with the capricious, reactive organization of standard neurotic womanhood.

Images of altruism and visionary idealism are presented as positive and healthy signs of social integration or spiritual aspiration. In contrast, the egoism and spiritual dreads which are symptomatic of Gwendolen's morbid consciousness, signal, in the broader framework of the novel, the potential for social and familial decline. In social terms, the relative insignificance of Gwendolen's small world is set against the vastness of history, the wider aspiration of Deronda, and the idealism of Mordecai:

---

[73] James Sully, *Sensation and Intuition: Studies in Psychology and Aesthetics* (London: Henry S. King, 1874), p. 87.

Could there be a slenderer, more insignificant thread in human history than this consciousness of a girl, busy with her small inferences of the way in which she could make her life pleasant?—in a time, too, when ideas were with fresh vigour making armies of themselves, and the universal kinship was declaring itself fiercely: when women on the other side of the world would not mourn for the husbands and sons who died bravely in a common cause, and men stinted of bread on our side of the world heard of that willing loss and were patient: a time when the soul of man was waking to pulses which had for centuries been beating in him unfelt, until their full sum made a new life of terror or of joy.

What in the midst of that mighty drama are girls and their blind visions?   (124)

Through the rhetorical paragraphing it is clear that Gwendolen's small life is inextricably bound up in the vaster movements around her, but these same movements impinge upon her consciousness in the form of terrifying manifestations of her own morbid vision. The 'mighty drama' is re-enacted as inner torment, in the 'recoil of her mind' (271) from any prospect of venturing from her small world into the unknown expanses beyond. In an image which is strikingly reminiscent of the delirious experiences of Dickens's Pip and Esther, Eliot describes Gwendolen's sense of dislocation from familiar points of reference. Finding herself alone amid wide horizons always 'impressed her with an undefined feeling of immeasurable existence aloof from her, in the midst of which she was helplessly incapable of asserting herself' (63–4), and she is seized with an agoraphobic terror which little by little crushes her 'lively venturesomeness' (271) into morbid imaginings of mental incarceration.

Gwendolen's internalization of external phenomena is in direct accordance with the symptomatology of 'morbid egoism' in which fear of nature's awesomeness is a characteristic sign of the distorted imagination that is incapable of unravelling or proportioning the range of possible meanings by inductive or deductive reasoning. Innocuous though this particular form of nervousness might seem, evolutionary physiologists construed it as a symptom not only of mental maladjustment but of arrested development. 'Everything appears supernatural when man knows nothing of the natural', wrote Maudsley in the introductory passages to his

Physiology of Mind. Whereas the healthy individual makes the appropriate 'internal adjustment to external impression', those of a more instinctual nature are more prone to allow sovereignty to subjective superstitions over objective knowledge.[74] The susceptible mind runs on dread of a phantasmagoric homogeneity of animate and inanimate entities, linking the sufferer in a pathological community with the primitive, the superstitious, and the believer in Divine, supernatural, and clairvoyant powers. Similarities between the self-centredness of neurosis and the 'self-concentration' of delirium are made evident in a register of morbid visions which unites Pip, Esther, Basil, and now Gwendolen in their loss of conscious control. In the opening chapter of *The Physiology of Mind*, Maudsley confidently attributes the origin of the fear of self-diminution in 'nature's vastness' to the inferior mental powers of humankind in the 'savage state of his infancy'. In the absence of ratiocination, writes Maudsley, the impressionable individual, governed by instinct and intuition rather than reason, 'falls down in an agony of terror' before the misunderstood forces which he wrongly believes to be directly, but unfathomably, associated with himself. These remarks were to shape a diagnosis which fitted conveniently with the evolutionary arguments for women's arrested intellectual development.

Although Gwendolen and Deronda acknowledge similar feelings of detachment and difference, their psychic experiences are dynamically distinguished as 'two lots [which] had come in contact, hers narrowly personal, his charged with far-reaching sensibilities' (621). While Gwendolen retreats into a terrifying world of ghosts, visions, and shadows, where her longings fragment and dissolve in ill-defined fantasies and short-lived sensations, Deronda's energies become 'an organic part of social life, instead of roaming in it like a yearning, disembodied spirit, stirred with a vague social passion' (365). The ghostly shadows which people Deronda's imagination are, unlike Gwendolen's, given a potential reality in the external world. Envisaged as

74 Henry Maudsley, *The Physiology of Mind*, rev. edn. of *The Physiology and Pathology of Mind* (London: Macmillan, 1876), p. 2. When G. H. Lewes addressed the question of the place of the supernatural in the civilized world, he too was adamant that scientific knowledge of natural laws would eventually eliminate belief in divine agency. *Problems of Life and Mind*, 3rd series, vol. 1. pp. 40–42.

veiled objects of the conscious search for his spiritual and familial roots, they represent for Deronda the fruits of rational
enquiry, and motivate an endeavour which is appropriate to the
single-minded resolve of male consciousness as opposed to the
alleged wavering impulsiveness of female imagination.
Deronda's will is the organizing force which channels his energies into constructive thought whereas, for Gwendolen,
nervousness has robbed her of a dominating will so that
thoughts and feelings have become confused in a twilight world
of undifferentiated dread. In the growing enmity following her
marriage to Grandcourt, Gwendolen's trepidation combines
with her troubled conscience about Lydia Glasher, her dislike of
Lush, her self-consciousness of Deronda's critical gaze, to
produce a dangerous compression in one 'schooled daily to the
suppression of feeling' (605):

The thought of [Grandcourt's] dying would not subsist: it turned as
with a dream-change into the terror that she should die with his throttling fingers on her neck avenging that thought. Fantasies moved
within her like ghosts, making no break in her more acknowledged
consciousness and finding no obstruction in it: dark rays doing their
work invisibly in the broad light.   (606)

The image of the 'dark rays doing their work invisibly in the
broad light' speaks once again both for science and superstition.
It accords with Lewes's physiological theory of the 'silent
growth of tendencies'—neural activity which operates beneath
the level of the will—and with unconscious thinking.[75] At the
same time, it hints at very unscientific ideas of demonic possession; superstitions which continue to instil fear, as Eliot earlier
observed, 'in an intense personality even in spite of theory and
science' (276).

If the physiological metaphor suggests, in relation to
Deronda, a potentiality for unity, an idea of a harmonious
system, for Gwendolen it denotes not unity, but a propensity for
malfunction. Looking outward, Deronda observes the world

---

[75] Sally Shuttleworth has pointed out that these ideas are consistent with Lewes's
arguments in relation to the 'Thinking Principle', in which he maintained that
consciousness was not of itself an agent, but merely a manifestation of a range of
activities and processes. See *George Eliot and Nineteenth-Century Science*, pp.
185–6.

and his part in it to be 'made up of plainly discernible links' (514) and it becomes his mission to identify the correct continuities between impression and idea, sensation and action. Conversely, Gwendolen's misinterpretation of the 'mighty drama' of external reality works against such comprehension. Her contrariness precludes the integration of self with the social environment and instead fragments that self into multiple ghostly presences imaged by Eliot as reflections of 'so many women petrified white' (359) in Lydia Glasher's diamonds scattered over the floor. Later, the urge to flee from the images that her own 'pent-up impulse' (673) has generated is intensified by the inescapable multiplication of her misery by the mirrors on board Grandcourt's yacht. The thematic and the psychological oppositions in the text set volition against impulse, autonomy against susceptibility, but they are not so securely established as to be able to define neurosis as irrevocably 'other' to a perceived norm. If, for instance, Gwendolen's waking dreams and heightened imagination are set against Mordecai's visionary idealism, their pathological status depends upon where the line between normal and diseased perception is drawn.

That very quandary was familiar to Eliot through the writings of Auguste Comte and more especially Claude Bernard. On the basis of a belief that the 'truth' of the normal can only be properly understood by studying the pathological, Bernard argued for their 'continuity' rather than their absolute difference. His dictum: 'Every disease has a corresponding normal function of which it is only the disturbed, exaggerated, diminished or obliterated expression' is dynamically different from models of polarity or obverse sides of the same coin.[76] Ideas of 'a struggle between two opposing agents, of antagonism between life and death, between health and sickness, inanimate and living nature have had their day', he asserts, and instead the 'continuity of phenomena, their imperceptible gradation and harmony must be recognized everywhere'.[77] Bernard's continuum thesis is

[76] *Lectures on Diabetes and Animal Glycogenesis* (Paris: J-B. Ballière, 1877), p. 56. Cited by Georges Canguilhem, *The Normal and the Pathological*, with intro. by Michel Foucault, trans. by Carolyn R. Fawcett (New York: Zone Books, 1989), p. 68.
[77] *Lectures on Animal Heat* (Paris: J-B. Ballière, 1876), p. 394. Cited by Canguilhem, *The Normal and the Pathological*, p. 72.

compatible with Lewes's view of objective facts and subjective response as the 'convex and concave surfaces of the same sphere'.[78] If disease was a relative not an absolute state, diagnosis becomes an interpretative skill which must take account of a whole range of variables, each shading imperceptibly into the next. The externalized visions of Mordecai and the internalized imaginings of Gwendolen are different dimensions ('convex and concave') of the continuum model of physiology and pathology.

In echoes of 'The Lifted Veil', Eliot raises the paradox of physical debility coinciding with heightened mental acuity. Mordecai is 'a consumptive-looking Jew' (471), whose 'ebbing physical life' coincides with a growing spiritual one. His visionary excitability, characteristic of the consumptive patient, expresses a yearning for spiritual perpetuation in another form. The sense of time running out generates the 'beneficent illusion' of the discovery of an 'expanded, prolonged self' (473), and the more the body decays, the more vivid are Mordecai's visions of a vital, healthy continuity projected, of course, onto Deronda. Mordecai preconceives Deronda out of the imagery of his own 'most passionate life' (479). If this form of prevision is to be regarded in the positive light of a necessary passion which 'even strictly-measuring science could hardly have got on without' (513) and, ultimately therefore, a sensible insurance against oblivion, it is undercut by the huge scientific question mark that Eliot places over the whole matter of premonition and clairvoyance. In an age of intellectual giants of positivism, the belief that all forms of engagement with the paranormal, including religious mysticism, were clear signs of hysterical neurosis was widespread.[79]

---

[78] *The Foundations of a Creed*, i. p. 112. The monistic philosophy of a reality consisting in a material convexity and an ideal concavity derives from Spinoza (d. 1677), on whom Lewes had written. Eliot refers to Spinoza in the same sentence as that in which Deronda attempts, with some difficulty, to interpret Mordecai from his sickly appearance alone (pp. 471–2).

[79] To note a few of the numerous examples: Robert Brudenell Carter, *On the Influence of Education and Training in Preventing Diseases of the Nervous System* (London: John Churchill, 1855), p. 227; George Edward Day, 'Louise Lateau: A Biological Study', Art.14, *Neurology*, [n.d.], 488–98. Lewes had a copy of this article; George H. Savage, *Insanity and Allied Neuroses: A Practical and Clinical Manual*, 4th edn. (London: Cassell, 1907), pp. 53–56; Henry Maudsley, *Body and Mind*, p. 85.

For Eliot, the contest between science and superstition is still to be decided. 'Second-sight', annunciates the narrator at the opening of Chapter 38, 'is a flag over disputed ground' (471).

Eliot's lengthy meditation on the much-disputed question of second-sight reopens the issue of diseased consciousness first explored in 'The Lifted Veil', but is here much less certain of the boundary between predictive fantasy and passionate vision. It interrogatively appropriates both the continuum model of Bernard and the demonic possession theory still insisted upon by George Duncan, whose evaluation of *The Various Theories of the Relation of Mind and Body* was among Eliot's and Lewes's books. If Duncan is right, spectral illusions are to be regarded as clear signs of incipient insanity. The question here seems to be whether there is a qualitative or a quantitative difference between Mordecai's obsession with the need for a spiritual heir, and Gwendolen's haunting by the picture in her mother's house of the 'upturned face' and the fleeing figure (27). What characterizes Gwendolen's obsession is her unassuageable dread that it is her morbid wish for Grandcourt's death that has given the impulse to her sick nerves to make thought spring into action. Here again, the 'dark rays' working within her are the manifestations of double consciousness; impulses allied to the imagination without the controlling influence of the intellect. These are not, however, unconscious nervous reflexes rooted in genealogy, but the re-animated terrors of a buried hatred. Originating in the innocent revelation of the opened panel, the images are overlaid with ominous significance so that they intensify into the 'hidden rites [which] went on in the secrecy of Gwendolen's mind' (673) and attach themselves to her consciousness of hatred and dread of her husband. Both 'spirits' (Mordecai's and Gwendolen's) are ultimately exorcized, the former through the continuity of embodiment in Deronda, and the latter through discontinuity, or more precisely, by means of Deronda's therapeutic severing of the causal links which Gwendolen has paranoically made between herself and external events.[80]

---

[80] For a different reading which argues for Gwendolen and Mordecai as types of the novel's two biblical and social worlds, see David Carroll, *George Eliot and the Conflict of Interpretations: A Reading of the Novels* (Cambridge: Cambridge University Press, 1992). Thomas P. Wolfe's 'The Inward Vocation: An Essay on

William Carpenter might well have been describing Gwendolen's inner turmoil when he writes of the way in which 'strange combinations' of 'fantastic and impossible creations' force themselves into the mind. In the 'internal tempest', he continues, false convictions are 'called into existence by external impressions, these being erroneously interpreted through the disordered action of the perceptive faculty'. In a dysfunctional nervous system, impulses of no especial significance become amplified into obsessional proportions, 'the mind having a tendency to *exaggerate* every impression made upon the consciousness, especially those which affect the emotional state'.[81] At different times, and for different reasons, obsession was constituted as a form of insanity and used as a measure of a person's capability of independent thought and sound judgement. One of these forms came to be known as 'monomania', described many years earlier by J. C. Prichard as 'a disorder of the mind in which a single false notion is impressed upon the understanding, which is otherwise unclouded, so that the insane person is capable of reasoning correctly on all subjects unconnected with a particular train of thought'.[82] However, in a treatise on medical jurisprudence, Prichard voiced some scepticism about whether monomania should be allowed to constitute a defence argument in criminal cases, pointing out that, although monomania had become established as a concept in the law, the notion of temporary, as opposed to partial, insanity had no medical foundation and could not excuse isolated acts of uncharacteristic violence. Despite these warnings, the idea of monomania gripped the public imagination and sensationalized many an enquiry into inexplicably violent or unsocial behaviour.[83] Clearly, the debates over monomania were still sufficiently alive

---

Daniel Deronda', *Literary Monographs*, 8 (1976), 1–46 offers a psychoanalytic reading of the relationship between Gwendolen and Deronda as does the rather less subtle Meg Harris Williams and Margot Waddell, *The Chamber of Maiden Thought: Literary Origins of the Psychoanalytic Model of the Mind* (London: Routledge, 1991).

[81] *Principles of Human Physiology*, p. 834, emphasis in original.

[82] *On the Different Forms of Insanity in Relation to Jurisprudence* (London: Hippolyte Ballière, 1842), p. 67. The theory of monomania was first formulated by J. E. D. Esquirol in *Mental Maladies: A Treatise on Insanity*, trans. by E. K. Hunt (1845; repr. New York: Hafner, 1965).

[83] Simon During has examined the moral implications of a possible 'localized but

in the 1870s to have a direct bearing on Eliot's disquisition on moral responsibility in relation to Gwendolen's mental health although, interestingly, her use of the term is applied to Mordecai rather than to Gwendolen. Deronda voices his concern about Mordecai's obsession as a 'suspicion that Mordecai might be liable to hallucinations of thought—might have become a monomaniac on some subject which had given too severe a strain to his diseased organism' (494). On the other hand, Gwendolen's consciousness of long desiring Grandcourt's death, and of her failure to act to save him from drowning, are ideas which converge in her mind only in the space of a moment. Ironically, it is the linking of unconnected impressions and events symptomatic of Gwendolen's sickness that is the very thing that exonerates her from blame, since it produces a narrative of remorse. But Gwendolen's admission 'I wished him to be dead. And yet it terrified me. I was like two creatures. I could not speak—I wanted to kill—it was as strong as thirst' (691) convinces Deronda that her guilt is of conscience and not of action. Henry Maudsley had spelled out the neurological distinction between irrational impulse and conscious volition in his treatise on insanity in *Body and Mind*, in a manner which seems to corroborate the legal one between intention and desire.[84] Eliot's awareness of these debates is reflected in her own enquiry as to where moral responsibility lies in matters of impulse. Although Deronda reasons that Gwendolen's murderous desires have not directly and inevitably turned to action, the question 'as to the outward effectiveness of a criminal desire dominant enough to impel even a momentary act' does not settle 'judgement of the desire' (696). In the perilous terrain of medico-legal designations of moral responsibility, Mordecai's consistency is shown to imitate the obsessive-compulsive behaviour of the

profound break in the unity of the psyche' in relation to the drowning incident in *Daniel Deronda* and the baffling case of Henriette Cornier, a servant girl who, in 1825, apparently without premeditation, decapitated the infant daughter of a local shopkeeper. This act subsequently became a precedent for monomania in criminal psychiatry. See 'The Strange Case of Monomania: Patriarchy in Literature, Murder in *Middlemarch*, Drowning in *Daniel Deronda*', *Representations*, 23 (1988), 86–104 (p. 86). On monomania, see also Jan Goldstein, *Console and Classify:The French Psychiatric Profession in the Nineteenth Century* (Cambridge: Cambridge University Press, 1987), chapter 5.

[84] *Body and Mind*, p. 71.

monomaniac, whilst Gwendolen's discontinuity and alarming compulsion to determine all outside objects towards the self are more closely allied to the rhetoric of hysterical neurosis.

Faced with the near-delirious 'confession' of the stricken Gwendolen, Deronda is reluctantly plunged into the role of the forensic psychiatrist called to adjudicate on the reliability of her statement. The quality of her evidence is undermined by the wretched state of her nerves which, as with Basil, Pip, and Esther, has rendered her unable to distinguish between dreaming and actual experience. In her disordered mind, the two merge into an interplay of phenomena of indeterminable status exemplified in the statement 'I only know that I saw my wish outside me' (696). Herbert Spencer had ascribed impressions devoid of the contexts which reflection or introspection give to them to 'inherited nervous organization'. Instead of marshalling feelings into their appropriate components 'within the experiences of the individual', the sufferer is so overcome by the torrent of intense, but 'vague and voluminous' impressions emanating from a distant and hitherto unrealized past, that the impulses produced out of that very formlessness become more vivid than those of immediate sentient life.[85] 'I saw my wish outside me' registers that confusion, but at the same time raises serious ethical questions of agency and responsibility. The split in Gwendolen's sense of autonomous selfhood recapitulates the theme of double consciousness and the conflicting narratives of the rational and the impulsive actor. It becomes Deronda's task to rearrange the disordered sense impressions into their proper categories, so severing the erroneous associations which her tormented mind has made between her malevolent thoughts and a chance event. Like Spencer, he reasons that the impressions produced out of the formlessness of the diseased consciousness have become more intense and affecting than those received from the material environment. Gwendolen's mistaken belief in the 'outward effectiveness' of her murderous wish to materialize into 'decisive action' is dismissed as a sick fantasy. This rationalization settles the hypothesis posited earlier in the novel that the mind can accommodate in one moment contrary feelings such as

---

[85] Herbert Spencer, *The Principles of Psychology*, 2 vols. (London: Williams and Norgate, 1855), i. pp. 579–608.

'the loyal and mean desire, for the outlash of a murderous thought and the sharp backward stroke of repentance', but contraries of action cannot be so accommodated for 'we cannot kill and not kill in the same moment' (42).

Interrogation of the mechanism that makes thought spring into action strikes at the very core of the neurological enigma. Maudsley had definite views on the registration of impressions and images upon the mind, and their subsequent recall. Though they lie dormant, they are never 'actually forgotten', he writes, 'no wave of oblivion can efface their characters.'

Consciousness, it is true, may be impotent to recall them; but a fever, a blow on the head, a poison in the blood, a dream, the agony of drowning, the hour of death, rending the veil between our present consciousness and these inscriptions, will sometimes call vividly back, in a momentary flash, and call back too with all the feelings of the original experience, much that seemed to have vanished from the mind for ever. In the deepest and most secret recesses of mind, there is nothing hidden from the individual self, or from others, which may not be thus some time accidentally revealed.[86]

Maudsley's term 'inscriptions' is crucial, it seems to me, to Eliot's depiction of Gwendolen's susceptibility to morbid impressions. It puts the connection between the incident of the opening panel which abruptly ended Gwendolen's performance of Hermione in Shakespeare's *The Winter's Tale* and the re-awakening of that incident following Grandcourt's drowning into a contemporary neurological context. Transfixed with terror that some malevolent force from the past had taken possession of her consciousness, Gwendolen's enactment of the quickening statue is curtailed by the horror of a sense of *déja vu* as much as by the image on the panel in itself. When, much later, overwhelming guilt revives the image of the dead face and the fleeing figure in her memory, that consciousness leads her to attach premonitory significance to the earlier incident and to believe its dreadful fulfilment in the second. The span of time between the two events collapses, as in delirium, and Gwendolen recalls how 'ever so long ago I saw it; and I wished him to be dead. . . . I felt beforehand I had done something

---

[86] *Body and Mind*, p. 21.

dreadful, unalterable—that would make me like an evil spirit. And it came—it came' (691). Indeed Deronda is so alarmed at Gwendolen's seeming inability to distinguish between external events and her own morbid thoughts that he is moved to ask himself: 'Was she seeing the whole event—her own acts included—through an exaggerating medium of excitement and horror? Was she in a state of delirium into which there entered a sense of concealment and necessity for self-repression?' (689).

To her observers, Gwendolen's susceptibility to impressions is symptomatic of her peculiar excitability, whereas, to her own mind, her terrors have been an embarrassing liability constituting 'an unexplained exception from her normal life' (63). But the notion of such attacks as mere inconveniences, as temporary aberrations from healthy life, is cast into doubt when Eliot accommodates Gwendolen's outbursts to the continuum hypothesis of pathology and to the evolutionary view of the 'silent growth of tendencies' linking fitful impressionability to a hereditary chain. Accordingly, these nervous dreads are construed not as indications of Gwendolen's especial sensitivity but as resurgences of 'a brief remembered madness'. An idea of ungovernable and ineradicable traces harboured in the nervous system is remarkably consistent not only with Maudsley's 'inscriptions' but with Lewes's proposition that residual impulses from the past 'count among the motors of the inner life'.[87]

Evolutionary medicine had found a way of including the isolated act, the 'brief madness' into hereditary constitution. Viewed in this new context, the acute stretched into the chronic and a whole range of otherwise unaccountable behaviour became amenable to diagnosis. Gwendolen's fits of terror correspond to Maudsley's attribution of brief madnesses to an underlying tendency to nervous disease which makes itself palpable in sudden and capricious displays, in violent seizure or cataleptic trance. 'In truth', he continues, 'nervous disease is a veritable Proteus, disappearing in one form to reappear in another, and, it may be, capriciously skipping one generation to fasten upon the next'. Maudsley's conviction that neurosis in the young is 'almost always traceable to nervous disease in the preceding

---

[87] *Problems of Life and Mind*, 3rd series, vol. 2, p. 97.

generation' seems pertinent when we note Eliot's narrator's allusion to 'a trace of demon ancestry—which made some behold-
ers hesitate in their admiration of Gwendolen' (68). But if Eliot
incorporated the paradigms of medical diagnosis into her narrative of physiological psychology, her study of Gwendolen's
gradual submission to the governance of her nerves does not
endorse those paradigms unequivocally. She believed that the
individual, like Lewes's organism, could not be accurately
understood without taking into consideration the social aspects
(or the organism's natural environment) of his or her life. The
interconnectedness of the psychological with the social is as
integral to *Daniel Deronda* as it was to *Middlemarch*, and
Eliot's intricate analysis of her heroine never loses sight of that
dimension.

In *Daniel Deronda*, conflict between the individual will,
desire, and expectation, and the overmastering forces of inheritance strikes at the very root of Gwendolen's identity. As she
emerges from childhood into adulthood, her sensitiveness is
construed as perversity and her aversion to physical contact as a
function of her own nervous dreads. Even her noted iridescent
quality suggests a conflict between the requirement to display her
eligibility and her simultaneous retreat from sexual commitment.
It is hardly surprising, she complains to Grandcourt, that when
women 'are brought up like the flowers, to look as pretty as we
can, and be dull without complaining,' like plants 'they are often
bored, and that is the reason why some of them have got poisonous' (135). The origins of Gwendolen's fear of intimacy are well
established. Even before her marriage to Grandcourt, we are told
that Gwendolen's idea of love was synonymous with an 'imaginative delight in being adored', and that she 'objected, with a
sort of physical repulsion, to being directly made love to' (70).
She embodies the ambiguity of sexual self-advertisement and
shrinking from physical contact, being at once 'the central object
of that pretty picture, and every one present must gaze at her'
(107) and 'subject to physical antipathies' when conscious of
being regarded by men for whom she did not care (122). Caught
in these bewildering contradictions, and tormented by
Grandcourt's cruelty, Gwendolen's responses are increasingly
extreme, ranging from paroxysmal outbursts to retreat into
silent suffering. The repugnance of proximity is the dread of

unwanted intrusion into the private space of the self; a dread that repeatedly manifests in the physical pain of strangling and suffocation familiar as 'globus hystericus', or the choking sensation of hysteria. Gwendolen's abhorrence of verbal confrontation with her husband slides, like a dream-change, into an anticipation of his 'throttling fingers on her neck' (565). In her fevered imagination, Grandcourt's indomitable will becomes the stranglehold of 'a crab or a boa-constrictor which goes on pinching or crushing' (423) and his words have 'the power of thumbscrews and the cold touch of the rack' (680).

While these images are the products of a morbid consciousness, they are also evocative of Eliot's implicit critique of contemporary theories of social development as unfailingly progressive. Nancy Paxton has argued that *'Daniel Deronda* presents a world where evolutionary processes seem somehow to have gone wrong, fostering tragic decay rather than "progress" ', a world in which marriage celebrates 'the triumph of will and ambition rather than mutual passionate love'. By creating a heroine whose emotional and sexual development has been 'curiously arrested', and who enters a 'murderous union defined by "negative" passions', Eliot is exposing what she considered to be serious flaws in social theories, principally those of Herbert Spencer, that were based on an unexamined use of Darwin's premiss of sexual selection.[88] For Eliot, then, biology in its raw state, as it were, cannot provide the key to a definitive anatomy of mental life or of the structure of society. As she shows in her portrayal of Gwendolen, observation alone may or may not reveal features and structures, but what those features and structures mean in terms of a functioning organism requires the more imaginative interpretation of the life science of physiology. Eliot brings the energies of that life science to bear on a study of the workings of the inner life which neither reduces them to neural functioning nor obscures them in a figurative landscape of mystic boundaries.

---

[88] Nancy Paxton, *George Eliot and Herbert Spencer: Feminism, Evolutionism, and the Reconstruction of Gender* (Princeton, NJ: Princeton University Press, 1991), pp. 202, 209.

CHAPTER FOUR

New Women and Neurasthenia: Nervous Degeneration and the 1890s

'ABERRANT PASSIONS, AND UNACCOUNTABLE ANTIPATHIES'

The last years of the century saw a hardening of the physiological arguments which had charged George Eliot's portrayal of psychological states. Theories of biological determinism, together with the supposed greater susceptibility of women to neuroses, produced a climate in which women's nervous illnesses were increasingly seen as the physiological consequence of their reluctance to comply with prescribed social and sexual roles. By the 1890s, women who were striving for more freedom from the constraints of domesticity were considered by many to be directly responsible for what was being presaged as the certain breakdown of the family as a social unit. Such women were regularly being warned by socio-medical commentators in journals and periodicals that they were doubly disadvantaged since they courted nervous illness if they resisted their biological destiny of marriage and motherhood, and were liable to give birth to weak and sickly children if they fulfilled it. The spectre of nervous degeneration loomed large over women's sexual lives as claims of inferior brain capacity and over-sensitive nervous organization called into question their constitutional fitness for the roles that nature and society had assigned them. It was not only medical men and sociologists, however, who endorsed the idea of a constitutionally morbid type. In an interview for *The Humanitarian*, the New Woman writer Sarah Grand, when asked her opinion of *Jude the Obscure*, commented: 'As for

"Sue", it would have been a good thing if someone had explained to her that she was not of the right constitution to marry. She was one of "Nature's Nuns", a morbid type that is being developed among us'.[1] Although Hardy would strenuously deny that Sue represented a 'type', the changes and developments in the years leading up to the end of the century nevertheless bore down on his portrayal of the heroine so as to compound her individuality with an implicit questioning of the institutional (social and scientific) structures responsible for bringing about those changes.

Sarah Grand had a point, however, inasmuch as Sue, not unlike Gwendolen Harleth in *Daniel Deronda*, harbours strong physical antipathies to a sexuality that is defined solely by the obligations of marriage and motherhood. Giving her own account of mental suffering experienced as physical pain, this equally 'fine-nerved, sensitive girl' confesses to Jude that Phillotson's presence is a torture to her:

Perhaps you have seen what it is I want to say?—that though I like Mr. Phillotson as a friend, I don't like him—it is a torture to me to live with him as a husband! . . . it is said that what a woman shrinks from in the early days of her marriage she shakes down to with comfortable indifference in half-a-dozen years. But that is much like saying that the amputation of a limb is no affliction, since a person gets comfortably accustomed to the use of a wooden leg or arm in the course of time! . . . But it is not as you think!—there is nothing wrong except my own wickedness, I suppose you'd call it—a repugnance on my part, for a reason I cannot disclose, and what would not be admitted as one by the world in general! . . . What tortures me so much is the necessity of being responsive to this man whenever he wishes, good as he is morally!—the dreadful contract to feel in a particular way in a matter whose essence is its voluntariness![2]

The sense of an inner private self that is at odds with an internalized expectation of external normality is unquestionably reminiscent of Eliot's Gwendolen. With a similar aversion to her

[1] Sarah A. Tooley, 'The Woman Question: An Interview with Madame Sarah Grand', *The Humanitarian*, ed. by Victoria Woodhull Martin, 8/3 (March, 1896), 160–9 (p. 169).

[2] Thomas Hardy, *Jude the Obscure* (1895), ed. by Patricia Ingham (Oxford: Oxford University Press, 1985), p. 223. Subsequent references to this edition will be given in the text.

husband's attentions, Hardy's heroine openly admits that her outwardly 'calm wedded life' is a lie, for, inwardly she is 'not really Mrs. Richard Phillotson, but a woman tossed about, all alone, with aberrant passions, and unaccountable antipathies' (215–16). Both women indicate a marked preference for the physical closeness of another woman but where, in Gwendolen's case, this is taken to be a sign of her immaturity, in the case of Sue, there is a knowingness about her own sexuality which is hinted at much earlier in the novel in the episode of the pagan statuettes.[3]

Sue's purchase of the naked figurines of Apollo and Venus, furtively smuggled into her chamber, presents a narrative of private passion and preoccupation which runs counter to her public image. After seeing Sue at work on her sacred texts, Jude assumes her to be 'steeped body and soul in church sentiment as she must be by occupation and habit' (93), an assumption quite contrary to Aunt Drusilla's view of such ecclesiastical commercialism as 'a perfect seed-bed of idolatry' (88). The discrepancy between Jude's idea of Sue's spirituality and her guilty secret—evidenced in her lying to Miss Fontover about her purchases and her perturbation at the sight of pagan nakedness next to her crucifix and Christian text—brings into focus a range of wider cultural discrepancies between female sexuality and desire, on the one hand, and patriarchal pronouncements on women's sexual and moral obligations, on the other. At a time when the life sciences were well established, biological explanations of sexual difference seemed to reinforce rather than banish old prejudices concerning mental powers and moral strengths.

Whereas in the first half of the century Auguste Comte's sociological complementarity of the sexes had idealized difference into harmonies of culture and nature, reason and feeling, evolutionary scientists were now adamant in asserting the subservience of the so-called female properties of 'nature' and 'feeling' to the male ones of 'culture' and 'reason'. Believing this hierarchy to be established in natural law, evolutionists accepted

---

[3] Gwendolen admits to her mother 'I can't bear any one to be very near me but you'. *Daniel Deronda*, ed. by Terence Cave (Harmondsworth: Penguin, 1995), p. 82. Sue makes a similar request to Mrs Edlin when she implores her to stay close by in an adjoining room while she re-consummates her marriage with Phillotson (416).

the idea of women's inferior mental capacity as fundamental. Many doctors and social commentators extended Darwinian theories into adjacent areas of research.[4] One of the areas against which a gender hierarchy of mental faculties was brought to bear was that of the predicted exhaustion of evolutionary energy. Amid the tensions raised by the findings of biologists and physicists in respect of nervous and global degeneration, old warnings about limited resources of energy were proclaimed with new conviction. The probability of degeneration at a cosmic level had been established at mid-century, when the second law of thermodynamics announced the slow but certain consumption of those precious resources. But the term 'degeneration' all too easily lent itself to psychological and moral interpretation. Bénédict-Augustin Morel's highly influential *Traité des dégénérescences physiques, intellectuelles, et morales de l'espèce humaine* had drawn attention, in 1857, to the apparent physical and mental deterioration in the younger generation of families, and given impetus to the belief that a process of regression or deviation from a once healthy standard was taking place. Defects, it was claimed, became exaggerated in the transmission from generation to generation or, more alarmingly, mutated to manifest in different forms in successive generations. Once the theories of female inferiority, finite energy, and nervous degeneration were considered together, it was not a huge step to the virtually unchallenged prognosis of mental and physical debility that attended those women who, increasingly in the last decades of the century, sought educational and economic equality with men.

Much of the fiction of the 1890s self-consciously engages with the physical and medical sciences, and with social and

---

[4] Whilst it is known that Darwin and Maudsley quoted from each other's work extensively, insights into the exchange of ideas among eminent thinkers are provided as much in correspondence as in published citations. For instance, the records of James Crichton-Browne, meticulously maintained during his tenure of office at the West Riding Pauper Lunatic Asylum in Wakefield (1866–76), refer to his correspondence with Charles Darwin, initiated by Henry Maudsley. See John Todd and Lawrence Ashworth, 'The House': Wakefield Asylum 1818–. . . . (Wakefield: the authors, 1993), p. 131. For a close study of the correspondence between Darwin and Crichton-Browne relating to their mutual interests, see Sander L. Gilman, *Seeing the Insane: A Cultural History of Madness and Art in the Western World* (New York: Wiley, 1982).

educational ideas to configure the new disease of 'neurasthenia', a nervous malady which came to be both causally and symbolically linked to the period. George Gissing's *The Whirlpool* and Thomas Hardy's *Jude the Obscure* are novels which situate narratives of nervous breakdown at the problematic intersection of biological theories of determinism and cultural anxieties about the alleged deleterious effects of modern life. The aim of this chapter is to look beyond the particulars of plot and personality which link these books thematically to New Woman fiction in order to reveal the extent of the influence of the biological and physical sciences in creating a culture of unease around the issue of sexual equality. Both novelists participate in the debates but position their respective heroines in different ways in relation to them. It might reasonably be argued that, as male-authored texts, *The Whirlpool* and *Jude the Obscure* are already in a dialogic, rather than uniform, relationship with New Woman fiction, in spite of Hardy's German reviewer who declared the representation of Sue to be 'the first delineation in fiction of the woman who was coming into notice in her thousands every year—the woman of the feminist movement'. It was a pity, however, the reviewer continued, that 'the portrait of the newcomer had been left to be drawn by a man, and was not done by one of her own sex, who would never have allowed her to break down at the end'.[5]

Scientific warnings about nervous degeneration and a general disquiet about the breakdown of the nuclear family engendered a sense of imminent crisis in the 1890s. Gissing's Alma Rolfe and Hardy's Sue Bridehead are studies in a form of nervous atrophy which many physicians directly related to this crisis. Undoubtedly, ambiguities in the medical literature which routinely listed both inherited degeneracy and over-refinement as contributory factors to nervous failure helped to foster a climate of fear. The nervous offspring of nervous families were condemned, or so it seemed, to inevitable degeneration, whether through the gradual winding down of deteriorating resources or the winding up of delicate nerves to breaking point. It was a gloomy outlook for those children whose 'systems lived on the

[5] Postscript, Preface to the 1st edn., p. xxxviii.

edge of dissolution' as fiction is ready to testify.[6] Demon ancestry is an ever-present determinant haunting texts, and the disastrous consequences of imprudent marriages are nowhere more hideously revealed than in *Jude the Obscure* where child murder and suicide raise the spectre of hereditary insanity manifesting itself at the end of a line of familial degeneration.

To add to the somewhat doom-laden aetiologies of nervous disease, the principle of an irrefutable link between the supposedly weaker female nervous system and woman's reduced mental capacity was proclaimed ever more vehemently. Again, social and sexual politics manipulated objective scientific fact and it scarcely needs saying that the seekers after emancipation continually came up against the might of establishment forces intent upon affirming women's natural subordination. Writings from across a range of disciplines addressed the particular issues of New Women, the marriage question, and modern life stress whilst indirectly subscribing to the general anxiety about biological degeneration and moral decline. When Hardy responded to questions put by the *New Review*, for instance, on the subject of sex education for girls before marriage, his fellow contributors included Sarah Grand, Walter Besant, Eliza Lynn Linton, the chief Rabbi, Hall Caine, and Max Nordau.[7] The intersection of ideas from the physical sciences, evolutionary biology, sociology, and neuropathology, together with social observation and simple sexual prejudice, fed a continuing debate on the nature and extent of the consequences of relaxing the divisions between the sexes. When scientists were called upon to ratify mental differences between men and women they were responding to growing fears that the present trend towards the erasure of difference would lead to social and moral turmoil.

In *The Descent of Man*, Darwin had pointed to woman's more strongly developed 'powers of intuition, of rapid perception, and perhaps of imitation', residual qualities that have carried over from 'a past and lower state of civilisation' as proof

[6] See George Frederick Drinka, *The Birth of Neurosis: Myth, Malady and the Victorians* (New York: Simon and Schuster, 1984) p. 100.

[7] Thomas Hardy, Art.VIII, 'The Tree of Knowledge', *New Review*, 10 (1894), 675–90 (p. 681).

of her under-developed higher faculties.[8] Herbert Spencer formulated his own ideas of sociology around evolutionary arguments relating to women's intellectual inferiority when, in *Principles of Sociology* (1876), he developed a rationalization of the ideal structure of the family according to which it was right and natural that women subordinated their intellectual activity to the necessary business of reproduction and nurture. 'We have seen', he announced, 'how the law of evolution in general, has been thus far fulfilled in the genesis of the family'.[9] The nuclear family is the highest achievement of evolution, but its harmony will only be maintained if the 'moral relations of married life' are founded on an acceptance of the essential difference between the sexes. Since there will always exist the need, he concludes, 'to compensate women for certain disadvantages entailed by their constitutions', the 'preponderance of power' must necessarily accrue to the husband 'as being the more judicially-minded' and possessing 'the greater massiveness of nature'.[10]

From the medical field, theory and practice endorsed separately gendered and culturally diverse physical and mental characteristics which, as now seemed certain, it had been the whole purpose of centuries of evolution to develop. Henry Maudsley repeated his evolutionist convictions with the authority of a moral philosopher:[11]

It is easy to distinguish two different classes of mind among mankind,—a subjective class marked by the tendency to feel intensely rather than to see clearly, or at any rate to mix feelings in observation and reasoning, more often met with amongst women than men; and an objective class, more able to look at things in the dry light of reason.

---

[8] Charles Darwin, *The Descent of Man, and Selection in Relation to Sex* (1871), 2nd edn. (London: John Murray, 1883), pp. 563–4.

[9] Herbert Spencer, *The Principles of Sociology* (1876), 3rd edn., 3 vols. (London: Williams and Norgate, 1904), i. p. 751.

[10] Ibid., i, p. 756.

[11] For studies of Henry Maudsley's career, see Trevor Turner, 'Henry Maudsley: Psychiatrist, Philosopher, and Entrepreneur', in W. F. Bynum, Roy Porter, and Michael Shepherd (eds.), *The Anatomy of Madness: Essays in the History of Psychiatry*, 3 vols. (London: Tavistock Publications, 1985), i, pp. 151–89; Michael Collie, *Henry Maudsley, Victorian Psychiatrist: A Bibliographical Study* (Winchester: St Paul's Bibliographies, 1988); and Daniel Pick, *Faces of Degeneration: A European Disorder, c. 1848–c. 1918* (Cambridge: Cambridge University Press, 1989), pp. 203–16.

It might fairly be argued that these different views of things are due to the relative predominance in consciousness of internal and external impressions, emotional persons having susceptible internal organs. Women at any rate appear to owe the self-feeling which shows itself in quick and mobile emotional susceptibility, in great part, to the cerebral sympathies of their reproductive organs.[12]

Alluding to what he termed the 'tyranny of their organization', Maudsley brought the plain statements of 'physiological fact' to bear upon women's susceptibility to nervous disorders, and to their disproportionate potential for sliding into more intractable mental disease.[13] In his frequently quoted article published in the *Fortnightly Review* in 1874, he brings together evolutionary, neurological, anthropological, and psychological theory to underline his warning that women who seek 'to contend on equal terms with men for the goal of man's ambition' do so at great peril to their nervous systems. The very different emotional natures of men and women can be traced back, he argues, to the dawn of the history of mankind, where they originated in the necessarily separate primitive instincts of 'self-preservation and propagation'. To attempt to iron out these essential differences is to try 'to undo the life-history of mankind from its earliest commencement'. 'Each sex must develope after its kind', he insists. Since marriage and motherhood are, and will continue to be, the first and foremost function of women, it stands to reason that their energies should be conserved for 'the peculiarities of their constitution, to the special functions in life for which they are destined, and to the range and kind of practical activity, mental and bodily, to which they would seem to be foreordained by their sexual organization of body and mind'.[14] The higher and more intricate faculties of thought and will, being properties of the more refined end of the evolutionary scale, are more properly the province of men.

The science which relegated women to a lower rank in the evolutionary scale received encouragement from another quarter

---

[12] Henry Maudsley, *The Physiology of Mind*, rev. edn. of *The Physiology and Pathology of Mind* (London: Macmillan, 1876), p. 377.

[13] 'Sex in Mind and in Education', *Fortnightly Review*, n.s. 15 (April, 1874), 466–83 (p. 468).

[14] Ibid., pp. 466, 470–1, 482.

when the autopsies carried out by James Crichton-Browne at the Wakefield Asylum affirmed that the female brain weighed approximately five ounces less than that of the male.[15] Predictably, much was made of what the physiologist George Romanes was later to label 'the missing five ounces of the female brain'.[16] For Crichton-Browne, a great admirer of Darwin, these findings seemed to confirm not only woman's inferior mental capacity but also a popular suspicion that, along with lunatics and primitive tribes, women were biologically determined to 'stop at a lower point in mental evolution'.[17] At the same time, the confused strands of scholarship which clustered around the preoccupation with mental difference between men and women led Crichton-Browne to concede that 'even from a medical point of view there is a good deal to commend in the higher education of women, for occupation of some kind is needful to save them from that dreary, aimless vacuity of mind that is hysteria's favourite soil'. But that occupation should not over-tax already limited resources. Girls and their guardians, he warned, are 'forgetful of the peculiarities of their organisation', and 'often study continuously like the other sex, and so induce depression, exhaustion, and irritability, and lay the foundation of many nervous derangements and occasionally of mortal diseases'.[18] Romanes attempts to settle the dispute once and for all by re-interpreting the term 'mental' according to the separate faculties which comprise it. An eminent evolutionary scientist, Romanes perhaps unwittingly exposes the dangers of drawing general truths from a single biological model and comes close to self-contradiction in an article which

[15] For studies of James Crichton-Browne, see Janet Oppenheim, '*Shattered Nerves': Doctors, Patients, and Depression in Victorian England* (New York: Oxford University Press, 1991), chapter 2; John Todd and Lawrence Ashworth, 'The House', pp. 115–50. In his diary for 1893, Hardy refers to 'an interesting scientific conversation' he had with Sir James Crichton-Browne from whom he learned that 'A woman's brain . . . is as large in proportion to her body as a man's', an unusual turn of phrase which avoids the absolute difference more often stressed. See F. E. Hardy, *The Life of Thomas Hardy 1840–1928* (London: Macmillan, 1962), p. 259.

[16] George J. Romanes, 'Mental Differences Between Men and Women', *Nineteenth Century*, 21 (1887), 654–72 (p. 666).

[17] James Crichton-Browne, 'Education and the Nervous System', in Malcolm Morris (ed.), *The Book of Health* (London: Cassell, 1884), pp. 269–380 (p. 342).

[18] Ibid., p. 312.

simultaneously proclaims that women's cerebral organization was arrested at a lower point in evolutionary development, and that their nerves had evolved to an over-refined delicacy and sensitivity. On the one hand, he ponders the insurmountable problems faced by the women currently seeking equal opportunities:

How long it may take the woman of the future to recover the ground which has been lost in the psychological race by the woman of the past, it is impossible to say; but we may predict with confidence that, even under the most favourable conditions as to culture, and even supposing the mind of man to remain stationary (and not, as is probable, to advance with a speed relatively accelerated by the momentum of its already acquired velocity), it must take many centuries for heredity to produce the missing five ounces of the female brain.[19]

And on the other, affirms woman's more advanced mental structure:

But if woman has been a loser in the intellectual race as regards acquisition, origination, and judgment, she has gained, even on the intellectual side, certain very conspicuous advantages. First among these we must place refinement of the senses, or higher evolution of sense-organs. Next we must place rapidity of perception, which no doubt in part arises from this higher evolution of the sense-organs—or, rather, both arise from a greater refinement of nervous organisation. . . . The whole organisation of woman is formed on a plan of greater delicacy, and her mental structure is correspondingly more refined: it is further removed from the struggling instincts of the lower animals, and thus more nearly approaches our conception of the spiritual.[20]

The contradiction between reversion and refinement becomes assimilated and endlessly repeated in many of the ideas which surfaced during the last years of the century.[21] It was centrally implicated both in medical case representations of nervous depletion and in the catastrophic experiences which blighted the lives of fictional characters in works of the period. Hardy plays on this very contradiction in portraying Sue Bridehead's nervous

[19] 'Mental Differences Between Men and Women', p. 666.
[20] Ibid., pp. 656, 660.
[21] For a discussion of the currency of theories of female inferiority and arrested development and their appeal to the Victorian establishment, see Cynthia Eagle Russett, *Sexual Science: The Victorian Construction of Womanhood* (Cambridge, Mass.: Harvard University Press, 1989).

collapse, as does Sarah Grand when she entitles Book 3 of *The Heavenly Twins* 'Development and Arrested Development'. Gail Cunningham has drawn attention to the 'heavy emphasis placed upon nervous disorder, disease and death' in almost all the fiction of the 1890s. In the novels both about New Women and by New Women writers, Cunningham remarks; '[m]ental breakdown, madness and suicide' are invariably the 'penalties the New Woman must pay for her attempts at emancipation'.[22] Gissing's *The Whirlpool* and Hardy's *Jude the Obscure* articulate, in different ways, the ideas which so preoccupied and troubled a generation. Published within a year of one another, their narratives are driven by the incompatibility of aspirations of progressive individuals and gloomy predictions of the degenerationists towards the seemingly inevitable catastrophe of nervous disintegration. *Jude the Obscure* is an archetypal text of the morbid interplay of impeded development and aspiring modernity. *The Whirlpool* contrives a metaphor for the deleterious effects wrought by modern trends, but it is more instructive for its inconsistencies and its over-simplified compartmentalizations as it strives to register and interpret those effects. This discussion concentrates on the portrayals of Sue Bridehead and Alma Rolfe, for it is the women in these novels whose nervous breakdowns are closely allied to the peculiarities of what Maudsley termed 'their sexual organization of body and mind'. Of course Hardy does not spare Jude from the crisis of contradictory forces that besets both protagonists, and Gissing only weakly and unconvincingly draws his hero Harvey Rolfe as one immune from the pressures which entice and finally overwhelm his wife. While both men's and women's disease was held, in some way, to be related to the conditions of the age, it was the exhausted bodies and ailing minds of women that were the indices of psychological and moral degeneration.

[22] Gail Cunningham, *The New Woman and the Victorian Novel* (London: Macmillan, 1978), p. 49. Cunningham points out that these disorder narratives emanate not exclusively from the pens of disgruntled men but from women writers such as Sarah Grand, Iota, George Egerton, Emma Frances Brooke, Mona Caird, and Ménie Muriel Dowie. Lyn Pykett sees the writing of Grand and other feminists as performing a more subversive function in their transposing of the terms of the contradiction to form a counter-ideology in which the brute nature of males placed them lower down in the evolutionary scale. *The 'Improper Feminine': The Women's Sensation Novel and the New Woman Writing* (London: Routledge, 1992).

Sarah Grand offers a different interpretation of the moral degeneration in families, but what Grand makes explicit about the progressive deterioration of families through the transmission of hereditary taint is implicit in Gissing's and Hardy's narratives.

Whether real or imagined, the pressures associated with the end of the century were registered in a new disease. Neurasthenia, or nervous exhaustion, excited a great deal of medical controversy centring, in the main, on the disputed contributory roles of heredity, gender, and modern life stress in its causation. Diagnosis of the disease enjoyed a vogue in England from the 1880s until the First World War, although British doctors were by no means unanimous in their recognition that this was an altogether new disease with a discrete clinical definition.[23] Clifford Allbutt voiced his doubts in a lengthy article in which he stated: 'I repeat that, like all other diseases, neurasthenia at its margins melts by infinite gradations into other morbid groups'.[24] Nevertheless, it served many a practitioner's need of a diagnostic category which would authorize the symptoms of fatigue as a clinical phenomenon and, in effect, encompass everything from listlessness to suicidal mania. It may well be the case that the cultural significance the disease acquired far exceeded the actual number of sufferers but, in important ways, neurasthenia was ideally suited to the concerns and preoccupations of the last decade of the century. It enabled both an explanation and a displacement of worrying symptoms by structuring an aetiology predicated on the contradiction between the rhetoric of progress and the statistics of declining health.

---

[23] The addition of 'neurasthenia' to medical history is customarily attributed to the American George Miller Beard, whose pronouncements on the pressures of modern life persuaded numbers of British medical practitioners that neurasthenia was indeed a new disease, whose causal criteria differed substantially from hysteria and hypochondriasis. Although Beard is generally credited with inventing the term, it had been independently used by another American, E. H. Van Deusen, an asylum superintendent who published a monograph on 'Neurasthenia' two months before Beard's article appeared. See John Chatel and Roger Peele, 'The Concept of Neurasthenia', *International Journal of Psychiatry*, 9 (1970–1), 36–49.

[24] 'Neurasthenia', in T. C. Allbutt and Humphry Davy Rolleston (eds.), *A System of Medicine*, 2nd edn., 9 vols. (London: Macmillan, 1905–11), viii, pp. 727–89 (p. 767).

Clifford Allbutt's remark on the amorphous contours of neurasthenia is significant. It is noticeable how slippery its defining criteria become when applied to men as opposed to women. While medical writers focus almost exclusively upon male breakdown from stress or over-work, novelists in England between the 1890s and the First World War typically associate the illness with the highly strung modern woman. In *The Whirlpool*, George Gissing makes a telling distinction between the declining health of Alma and the condition of the metropolitan male. Around the time that Gissing was writing *The Whirlpool*, Thomas Stretch Dowse, a physician outspoken on the connection between modern civilization and ill health, is adamant that the anxiety brought on by the relentless drive to succeed in a frenetic modern world was draining men of their natural resources of strength.[25] Dowse, like Gissing, subscribed to the evolutionist view that mental and physical potential was already determined according to kind. The work of both men confirms and validates sexual (as well as class and racial) difference by means of narratives which asseverate the morbid consequences of living beyond one's biological means. In Britain, the new disease of nervous exhaustion was considered, theoretically, to be non-sex-specific, yet the medical literature concentrated almost exclusively upon male cases, where justifiable cause was much easier to ascertain. Men whose professional or business lives exposed them to financial and ethical stresses from which women were mostly protected were more liable, it was argued, to be struck down by a disease involving the wear and tear of complex vital structures. Dowse draws his case histories almost exclusively from the crushed man of business, the erstwhile tireless 'strong, athletic, active man, with nerves like iron bands', who now, as a result of stretching himself too far, has become 'chained and shackled by the demon neurasthenia'. It is 'foolish and puerile', he insists, to dismiss this enervating disease as mere nervousness.[26] When Gissing remarks on the 'grizzled, scraggy-throated, hollow-eyed' appearance of the

[25] Dowse's views are set out in *On Brain and Nerve Exhaustion (Neurasthenia), and on the Nervous Sequelæ of Influenza* (London: Baillière, Tindall, and Cox, 1894).

[26] *On Brain and Nerve Exhaustion*, pp. 27–8.

metropolitan male, he is unequivocally linking his physical deterioration to the strain of modern life in general, and to the collapse of the Britannia Loan, Assurance, Investment, and Banking Company in particular.[27]

On the other hand, the diagnosis and treatment of women sufferers more typically addressed the individual psychological make-up of the patient rather than external causes. Consequently, studies of female nerve exhaustion were invariably veiled criticisms of an unstable will and personal moral weakness. Practitioners who treated neurasthenia in women often regarded it in the light of a moral visitation upon reckless individuals who ignored warnings about the perils of physical or mental excess.[28] In my labelling of Alma Rolfe and Sue Bridehead as 'neurasthenic', it is in the knowledge that the narratives of their ailing health have as much to do with the ideological inconsistencies around which the disease was formulated as with a definitive pathology. The novelistic depictions of nervous exhaustion by Gissing and Hardy are informed by the continuing debates on the New Woman and the pressures of modern life, but are suffused with something more sinister. In stark contrast to the languid, drawing-room face of neurasthenia associated, in some minds, with over-worked, over-conscientious professionals or intellectually under-worked housewives was the hereditary degeneracy factor which, importantly, held a morbid fascination for the authors of *The Whirlpool* and *Jude the Obscure*. Fears of nervous degeneration on a massive scale, not helped by the 'whirlpool' of modern life, had been gathering momentum in the wake of evolutionary theories of descent. The belief that a predisposition to nervous susceptibility was inherited from ancestors who may or may not have been neurotic, but were

---

[27] George Gissing, *The Whirlpool* (1897), ed. by Patrick Parrinder (London: Harvester, 1977), p. 6. Subsequent references to this edition will be given in the text.

[28] It is worth noting that the notoriously contentious 'rest cure' treatment devised by Silas Weir Mitchell, a compatriot of George Miller Beard, never achieved quite the cult status it had in America since sceptics believed that it prolonged, confirmed, and endlessly redefined the neurasthenic in the very sickness it purported to cure. The dubious benefits of the rest cure were the target of feminist criticism even at the time, most notably in the American short story 'The Yellow Wallpaper' by Charlotte Perkins Gilman. Criticism was principally on the grounds that it was open to abuse by conspiratorial husbands and doctors attempting to silence and shackle wilful or restless wives and patients.

certainly defective, organically, mentally, or morally, conjoined with physical laws of finite energy, and the phenomenon of urban and industrial expansion, to foster the idea of biological degeneration.

Much of the fiction of the period stands as a testimony to the bleak nihilism that ideas of biological degeneration provoked in the imagination. For Hardy especially, the growing awareness that the subtle complexities of the human spirit seemed to become meaningless and purposeless in the shadow of the scientific laws of the universe only hardened his pessimism. When, in the Preface to the first edition of *Jude the Obscure*, he explains his attempt to communicate the austerity of life's 'deadly war waged between flesh and spirit' and its 'tragedy of unfulfilled aims', his words are heavy not only with a cultural despair of institutions but with a sense of a human race tending towards physical, mental, and spiritual asthenia.[29] Theories of diminishing resources, at both individual and cosmic levels, proliferated in the latter part of the century and found a deal of supporting evidence in alarmist interpretations of observed trends. Everything from a general malaise to epilepsy to insanity came to be re-examined according to degrees of degeneration along a sliding scale from the 'normal' to the 'abnormal'.[30] Max Nordau's book *Degeneration*, first published in 1892, exercised a pernicious and pervasive influence by proclaiming a connection between hereditary degeneration and the spiritual and moral decadence he claimed to observe in contemporary art and literature.[31] The term 'degeneration' was never free of moral connotations and it became a central image in the literature whose plot concerns were the perceived crisis in the institution of the family, whether brought about by feminist rebellion or, as in Ibsen's play *Ghosts* or Grand's *The Heavenly Twins*, by the transmission of degenerative disease through sexual sin. In the knotty contexts of marriage and emancipation, of family and sexuality, degeneration lurked ominously in the consciousness as an oppressively physiological determinant which threatened to render all other discourse futile.

[29] *Jude the Obscure*, p. xxxv.
[30] See Francis Schiller, *A Möbius Strip: Fin-de-Siècle Neuropsychiatry and Paul Möbius* (Berkeley: University of California Press, 1982), pp. 74–5.
[31] Max Nordau, *Degeneration* (1892), trans. from 2nd edn. (London: Heinemann, 1913).

It is this conformation of ideas which helped to fashion neurasthenia as an illness which lent itself to medical alarmism and moral panic. In a general sense it became bound up with the blurring of gender roles which was a feature of *fin de siècle* culture and, strangely, in view of the published medical evidence, associated with the spectre of the New Woman and the supposed threat to social and sexual stability that the emancipated woman was deemed to constitute. The presence of such sexually ambiguous figures as the New Woman, the dandy, and the aesthete in what Elaine Showalter, borrowing from Gissing, has called the 'sexual anarchy' of the *fin de siècle* was indicative of the confusion of roles.[32] In *Jude the Obscure*, the narrator invokes the classical image of gender ambiguity in homoerotic art to describe Sue, dressed in Jude's great-coat, as 'boyish as a Ganymedes' [*sic*] (159). Sarah Grand develops the image of gender ambiguity much more fully to raise cultural questions about the construction of gender division in childhood and education. Angelica, who cross-dresses in her brother Diavolo's clothes in order to experience life as a man, is astonished to find that so slight a change immediately gives her the intellectual and social freedoms she is denied as a woman. It is impossible not to be struck by the similarity between Sue Bridehead's disclosure to Jude of having mixed with men 'almost as one of their own sex. I mean I have not felt about them as most women are taught to feel—to be on their guard against attacks on their virtue' (152) and Angelica's observation to the man known as the tenor: 'Had you known that I was a woman ... the pleasure of your companionship would have been spoilt for me, so unwholesomely is the imagination of a man affected by ideas of sex'.[33]

For most of *Jude the Obscure*, Jude and Sue struggle and spectacularly fail in their attempt to lay out, and live by, a new set of ground rules designed to free them from what they see as

[32] Elaine Showalter, *Sexual Anarchy: Gender and Culture at the Fin de Siècle* (London: Virago, 1992), p. 3.

[33] Sarah Grand, *The Heavenly Twins* (1893), ed. by Carol A. Senf (Michigan: University of Michigan Press, 1992), p. 458. Subsequent references to this edition will be given in the text. For an interesting analysis of this episode which draws attention to parallels between Grand's writing and that of the male Decadent in respect of a marked desire to overturn fixed sexual identities, see Sally Ledger, *The New Woman: Fiction and Feminism at the Fin de Siècle* (Manchester: Manchester University Press, 1997).

the intellectually and spiritually repressive constraints of social and biological expectation. Gissing's Alma and Harvey Rolfe are more pragmatic in formulating their principles but scarcely more successful in carrying them out. Their tentative reversal of roles—Alma's public engagements and Rolfe's management of the nursery and Hughie's education—signals their emancipation and enlightenment even as it precipitates their dissolution. Rolfe feels uncomfortable in the man's world of finance, dealing, and speculation, considering it to be akin to meddling 'shamefaced, into the secrets of an odious vice' (208). But, at the same time, it is somewhat grudgingly that he acknowledges to Hugh Carnaby how the 'days are past when a man watched over his wife's coming and going as a matter of course. We should only make fools of ourselves if we tried it on. It's the new world, my boy; we live in it, and must make the best of it' (215). Harvey Rolfe's albeit grudging acceptance of changing times, and his genuine concern that his son's education should be different from his own, point to Gissing's engagement in the debate on the shifting dynamics of the family. In *Jude*, it is through Phillotson that Hardy addresses the implications, for men, of women's bid for autonomy when, after Sue has abandoned him to return to Jude, he voices his respect for her principles to his less-charitable friend Gillingham. Even more radically, Phillotson counters Gillingham's alarm that allowing women to do as they please will result in the disintegration of the family unit with the view that women and children form the new family, there being no more need of men as patriarchal overlords.

If Gissing has Alma suffer for her modern ideas, Hardy has Sue suffer on account of society's unpreparedness for the cultural changes that her principles envisage. In Sarah Grand's *The Heavenly Twins*, the case for a radical change in attitudes to marriage is put unhesitatingly at the door of sexual behaviour and the suffering that some women endure because of society's acceptance of a double standard for men and women. Grand mildly rebukes Hardy for not being outspoken enough on the matters of marriage and morals. His book is ethically evasive, Grand holds, and tends no further than to show how 'erratic relations between the sexes result in misery'.[34] For Hardy, of

34 *The Humanitarian*, p. 169.

course, the misery was not solely the direct result of erratic relations but a consequence of the powerlessness of the human spirit and human aspirations in the face of overwhelming social and biological forces. Grand has a different agenda and the frankness with which *The Heavenly Twins* approaches the subject of men's and women's sexual lives brings the burning issue of health and heredity into the forefront of debate. Dissolute behaviour, Evadne tells Mrs Orton Beg, cannot be overlooked and banished to the past for 'there is no past in the matter of vice. The consequences become hereditary, and continue from generation to generation.'[35] It is, perhaps, unsurprising that neither Gissing nor Hardy puts male sexual depravity at the centre of their narratives but the preoccupation with the modern woman, health, heredity, and the future of the family is a predominant literary and cultural imperative.

If the collective anxiety generated by these coincident preoccupations was the incentive for designating a disease of modern life, in a paradoxical way, it was the very vagueness and versatility of such a disease which worked to dissociate its depressive symptoms from the more terrifying neurological and psychological signs that bore the stamp of hereditary degeneracy. This dissociation, however, did not stop either clinical or fictional narratives of neurasthenia from scrutinizing ancestry for clues to an individual sufferer's defects of stamina and mental or moral powers. Since the 1870s, as was noted in a previous chapter, Darwinist doctors and psychiatrists had become alerted to the significance of ancestral traits as a scientific, not just a moral, consideration in their patients' neuroses. But until knowledge of genetics began to explain the mechanism of heredity, the appearance of atavistic traits was viewed with a superstitious terror.

Atavism or reversion seemed to be a further reminder of the powerlessness of the individual consciousness when set against the inexorable laws of biological science. When overlaid with moral significance, this unpalatable notion became intertwined with the numbers of other disconcerting phenomena of the day, including that of the New Woman. Grant Allen, whose popular novel, *The Woman Who Did*, is frequently cited as typifying a

---

[35] *The Heavenly Twins*, p. 80.

short-sighted male confusion of women's desire for social, legal, and professional independence with a perceived sexual licentiousness, uses the hereditary model as a warning to aspiring female consciousness. According to its terms, progressive ideas in one generation will only lead to a reversion to ancestral type in the next. The disappointment of his Girton-girl heroine, Herminia Barton, in her commonplace and conventional daughter Dolores, leads Herminia to despair at the failure of her endeavour, and she commits suicide by taking prussic acid. The reign of the virago New Woman seems destined to collapse with the reassertion of a primitive simplicity in her offspring. Since Dolores's upbringing had been anything but commonplace and traditional, her opinions, writes Allen, must have come from within by 'pure effort of atavism'. 'Heredity of mental and moral qualities', he adds, 'is a precarious matter'. Though Herminia's daughter had been exposed only to the most radical and liberating ideas, 'she herself seemed to hark back, of internal congruity, to the lower and vulgarer moral plane of her remote ancestry'.[36] In *The Whirlpool*, Gissing seems concerned with the more direct transmission of morbid traits from parents to children as being indicative of an irreversible downward trend. The preoccupation with hereditary degeneracy is introduced early in the novel when Mrs Abbott tries to interest Rolfe in Ribot's *L'Hérédité psychologique*, a book which has clearly influenced her assessment of the Wager children presently in her care. Shocked by their vulgarity, Mrs Abbott sneeringly remarks: 'What could one expect with such a father?', but then, somewhat inconsistently, blames their street-talk and low-class behaviour on their father's abandonment of his 'luckless brats' to their fate (29).

While Hardy avoids the crude moralizing of Allen and Gissing, both his *Jude the Obscure* and Gissing's *The Whirlpool* cite defective ancestry as the crucial component in their protagonists' inability to cope with the demands of the present. For novelists well read in matters of heredity, it would have been axiomatic that knowledge of one's forebears held the key to an individual's vital reserves, and to the capacity for withstanding adversity or collapsing under it. A point that was constantly

---

[36] Grant Allen, *The Woman Who Did* (London: John Lane, 1895), pp. 191–3.

laboured in scientific tracts was that defects in one generation prenatally diminished the vital reserves of the next. Typically, when Dowse affirmed that '[i]n neurasthenia . . . defective will power, defective resisting power, defective memory, defective power of application and attention, and not unfrequently the special senses are defective and perverted; *perversion really reigns supreme*', he was at pains to point out that, unlike mere nervousness, the severity of the depletion came at the end of a long line of cumulative degeneration.[37] Moreover, by 1894, many physiologists would have agreed with Dowse that inherited constitution was not simply the inheritance of 'blood or tissue elements' but much more subtly of 'mental states and nerve forces' which may present in one form in one generation but may find a different seat of location in the next.[38] Evidence of familial decline was not hard to find, and the model of transmission set out by Bénédict-Augustin Morel in his *Traité des dégénérescences* still carried authority. It was widely feared that succeeding generations became progressively weaker, with defects being compounded so that what may have begun as nervousness led to neurological disease in the next, psychosis in the third, to be followed, in turn, by idiocy and death.[39]

The bleak logic of progressive deterioration appealed to those who, like Hardy, could conceive of no respite from Darwinian physiological determinism. Peter Morton has suggested that when Hardy came across August Weismann's *Essays Upon Heredity* in 1890, he discovered in its pages confirmation of his own unremitting nihilism.[40] Weismann's assertion that an

[37] Thomas Stretch Dowse, *On Brain and Nerve Exhaustion*, p. 27, emphasis in original.

[38] *On Brain and Nerve Exhaustion*, pp. 40–2 (p. 41). Dowse's observation was not altogether new. In his book *Sensation and Intuition: Studies in Psychology and Aesthetics* (London: Henry S. King, 1874), James Sully concurred with Darwin and Spencer in recognizing the transmission of impulses and habits as well as physical traits. See Gillian Beer, *Darwin's Plots: Evolutionary Narrative in Darwin, George Eliot and Nineteenth-Century Fiction* (London: Ark Paperbacks, 1985. First published 1983), p. 215.

[39] For a much fuller discussion of the influence of degeneration theory in literature and the wider culture, see William Greenslade, *Degeneration, Culture and the Novel 1880–1940* (Cambridge: Cambridge University Press, 1994).

[40] August Weismann, *Essays Upon Heredity and Kindred Biological Problems*, 2 vols. (Oxford: Clarendon Press, 1889–92). For the reference to Hardy's reading in 1890 see F. E. Hardy, *The Life of Thomas Hardy*, p. 230. For an account of

immutable 'germ plasm' passed from generation to generation strengthened Hardy's belief in the tyranny of biology and the delusion of individual aspiration in all areas of mental, moral, and spiritual life. As far as Hardy was concerned, the most disturbing aspect of the germ plasm theory was that it posited a mechanism of transmission which operated independently and uninfluenced by the experiential life of the organism it inhabited. If Weismann were to be believed, the body was merely a conduit for the germ plasm. When Hardy writes, then, of Sue Bridehead's grandiose schemes of spiritual freedom and intellectual independence, her naive optimism is already underwritten with her creator's conviction that such self-determined consciousness was inherently at odds with the evidence of science.

Gissing shows scant sympathy for his New Woman's acts of emancipation from preordained marital and sexual structures and, like the vast majority of commentators on the morbid familial consequences of such acts, interprets them as signs of aberrance. *The Whirlpool* draws much more heavily than does Hardy's *Jude* upon the tenuous pronouncements about the inadequacy of women to perform anything other than the reproductive, nurturing, and affective roles for which, it is alleged, they have been biologically destined. Alma's neurasthenia is represented as the consequence of recklessness, of a refusal to heed the warnings of a scientific patriarchy. Sue Bridehead's neurasthenia is more complexly configured. Her fine intellect and sensitivity speak without question to the consciousness of the period. But, at the same time, her neurasthenia is specific to her individual organization, more a matter of temperament than type. The attitudes she strikes are not so much acts of purposeful resistance as the only ones possible in a woman neurologically unfitted for the roles of marriage and motherhood. Not that that excuses her in the judgement of the narrator whose observations barely conceal the suggestion that Sue's antipathies are self-generated:

Weismann's influence on Hardy, see Peter Morton, *The Vital Science: Biology and the Literary Imagination, 1860–1900* (London: Allen and Unwin, 1984), pp. 198–204.

Then the slim little wife of a husband whose person was disagreeable to her, the ethereal, fine-nerved, sensitive girl, quite unfitted by temperament and instinct to fulfil the conditions of the matrimonial relation with Phillotson, possibly with scarce any man, walked fitfully along, and panted, and brought weariness into her eyes by gazing and worrying hopelessly.   (229)

Alma's recklessness and Sue's over-refined sensitivity are indicative of the different emphasis that the two novelists placed upon the neuropathic conditions affecting England at the end of the nineteenth century. On one of those conditions, they seemed to be in agreement.

The disease of neurasthenia was very pointedly distinguished from other forms of neurosis by its precipitation by the strains of modern life. Industrialization, urban expansion, the mechanization of the workplace, and the railways were variously or collectively blamed for producing the phenomenon of nervous exhaustion. 'Life at high-pressure', exhorted Dowse 'is the prominent feature of the nineteenth century, and we cannot be surprised when we find that the so-called nervous diseases and exhaustions, dipsomania and insanity, are increasing beyond all proportion to the rapid increase of the population'.[41] 'Life at high pressure' is precisely Harvey Rolfe's trenchant response to Alma's report of her father's frenetic daily round (40). Hardy had made notes on the neuropathic effects of the 'fiendish precision or mechanism of town-life' around the time he was contemplating a plot which was to grow into *Jude the Obscure*.[42] In his novel, the link between nervous disease and modern life, if not as central as in *The Whirlpool*, is nevertheless implicit. All of the main characters are in various stages of transit, deracinated from the culture of their forebears and driven by the imperative to adapt to something new. The narrative's itinerant leaps between Marygreen, Christminster, Melchester, Shaston, Aldbrickham, and Elsewhere reflect in large scale the mental or physical restlessness of the individuals who find few points of fixity for their attainments or aspirations. A sense of life speeding up is both immanent and everywhere apparent. Sue herself remarks on how the railway station

[41] *On Brain and Nerve Exhaustion*, p. 51.
[42] *The Life of Thomas Hardy*, p. 207.

has supplanted the cathedral as the hub of town life (139). And it is Sue's transplantation from the quiet backwater of Marygreen to the city that is more than once offered as the reason for her quivering modernity. Aunt Drusilla predicts the disastrous consequences of the combination of a nervous disposition and town life when she warns Jude that his cousin was always a 'pert little thing . . . with her tight-strained nerves', but if she has now grown 'townish and wanton it med bring 'ee to ruin' (113–14).

Townishness is the pejorative epithet which condemns Alma Rolfe and many other female figures in *The Whirlpool* to a pathological status. Gissing's 'whirlpool' metaphor maintains the association between disease and urban life throughout the novel by signifying at once the vortex that is fashionable metropolitan society and the swirling pit of individual psychic turmoil in which those who choose to live life at high pressure are ultimately consumed.[43] It was, as I shall later show, a matter of some contention whether modern life could, of itself, cause nervous collapse. To informed minds the 'vertigo and whirl of our frenzied life' to which Nordau subscribed could only accelerate or aggravate an already defective organization.[44] Both hereditary and acquired factors had long been considered in the diagnosis of nervous disease, as has often been noted. George Gissing's *The Whirlpool* exploits the modern life stress elements of neurasthenic decline while continually reminding us of the pressure of heredity by locating the source of Alma's illness in her reckless disregard for ancestral weakness. The preoccupying issues of the day, notably the New Woman, degeneration theory, social change, sexual anarchy, and nervous disease, all charge its pages, but, unlike *Jude the Obscure*, the result is a disconcerting rather than tragic depiction of physiological degeneration and psychopathological determinism.

---

[43] Gissing purposely names his hero after William Harvey, the physician who discovered the circulation of the blood, *c.* 1651. See *The Whirlpool*, p. 120.
[44] *Degeneration*, p. 42.

REBELLION AND RECKLESSNESS IN *THE WHIRLPOOL* OF MODERN LIFE

As most critics have pointed out, it is Gissing's heroine, Alma Rolfe, who embodies the cultural anxieties and ideological tensions of the age in her frenzied pursuit of self-fulfilment outside the allotted sphere of maternal domesticity. Brought up in a prosperous, middle-class family, Alma's expectations of a comfortable life with independent means are shattered when her father, Bennet Frothingham's, banking and investment company collapses, and he commits suicide. Alma is then faced with a choice between marrying for a secure and respectable life of domesticity or earning her own living. Like Sue Bridehead, Alma aspires to be a free spirit, but, like Hardy's heroine, she has no clear idea of how that might be achieved, particularly within the context of Victorian marriage. Her marriage to Harvey Rolfe promises material comforts and social ease which make her envisaged career as a concert violinist unnecessary in survival terms, with the result that her desire for eminence in that sphere dissipates into the self-limiting success of drawing-room culture. Despite a commendable search for fixity through the development of rewarding relationships, Alma merely flits from scheme to scheme until she finds herself alienated both from the idealism of the domestic tranquillity of early married life in a country retreat and the pretentious superficiality of the metropolitan whirl. Little by little, Alma is sucked into a world of intrigue, fear, and secrecy. No longer in control of events or of her responses to them, she takes solace in ever-increasing doses of what Gissing euphemistically refers to as her 'draught of oblivion', her 'remedy for insomnia' (448). Alma's taking of her own life is dismissed with indecent haste by a doctor who rules, in a peremptory manner, that she had been warned, and by a final chapter which effectively draws a veil over her very existence.

My reading of the novel is not so much a pointing up of Gissing's often bitter and complicated misogyny, but an exploration of the way in which the specific beliefs, attitudes, and fears of the 1890s were incorporated into a case study of the neurasthenic Alma Rolfe. From the start, Alma's passion for an independent, self-determined life is undercut with imputations of foolhardy rebelliousness:

About the middle of December, Alma Frothingham left England, burning with a fever of impatience, resenting all inquiry and counsel, making pretence of settled plans, really indifferent to everything but the prospect of emancipation. The disaster that had befallen her life, the dishonour darkening upon her name, seemed for the moment merely a price paid for liberty. The shock of sorrow and dismay had broken innumerable bonds, overthrown all manner of obstacles to growth of character, of power. She gloried in a new, intoxicating sense of irresponsibility. She saw the ideal life in a release from all duty and obligation—save to herself.   (66)

The implicit reproach sets the tone of narratorial comment on Alma throughout the novel. But the cultural paradoxes of *fin de siècle* representation produce an ambiguous narrative in which few escape physical or psychological impairment as a direct consequence of their lifestyle. Rolfe admits that the problem they all face in a civilized society is a 'general failure of energy' which he has known himself intermittently 'only too well' (166). And yet Alma's fluctuations between manic activity and utter exhaustion are attributed to a peculiarly feminine mental incapacity to regulate her life. Her inability to withstand the lure of fashionable society or to see it for what it is worth is put down to constitutional weakness and gradually, but inexorably, she is drawn towards the contaminating source of social and individual devitalization. At the close of the novel she is simply written out; an unmourned casualty of a life of intrigue, passionate excess, and recklessness.

The Whirlpool has been described as a novel replete with 'over-refined women and atavistic men', but yet in which authorial sympathy clearly aligns with Harvey Rolfe.[45] Rolfe takes it upon himself to interpret Alma's decline in accordance with current opinion on the dangerous combination of inherited weakness and the misplaced expenditure of energy in the public sphere. But the men and women in this novel cannot be so neatly categorized as Parrinder's summary would suggest. It is difficult, for example, to square Rolfe's observation of the

---

[45] Patrick Parrinder, Introduction, p. xxii.

way 'that women came up from supper with flushed cheeks
and eyes unnaturally lustrous. What a grossly sensual life was
masked by their airs and graces!' (41–2) with a view of their
over-refinement. On the other hand, male atavism is contra-
dicted by Rolfe's ready, if not altogether willing, acknowledge-
ment of a shifting gender hierarchy. Giving nominal support to
his wife's projects, he insists that he does not wish her to be
'dutiful and commonplace' (168). It was agreed, he reminds
her, that 'you're not to subordinate your life to mine. That's the
old idea, and it still works well with some people. . . . At all
events, it won't work in our case' (167–8). As the story of
Alma's bid for personal fulfilment unfolds, Rolfe's magnani-
mous gestures of liberal-mindedness turn sour in the gulf of
jealousy, suspicion, and mistrust which opens up between
them. Far from rejoicing in Alma's nervous energy, talent,
attractiveness, and vitality, Rolfe begins to inspect these same
qualities for signs and symptoms of nervous degeneration.
Gissing's representation of Alma's mounting troubles, though
without doubt medically informed, presents a less-settled
picture of the causes and effects of female neurosis than the one
he tries to paint. With its contrived aetiology and uncertain
boundaries, the disease of neurasthenia could contain the paradoxes of atavism and refinement, cultivation and degeneration,
enabling a discourse of ambivalence which both inspired and
perplexed a generation of writers and thinkers from scientific
and literary fields.

To the extent that Gissing was influenced by his reading of
Nordau's *Degeneration*, as critics have argued, his reproduction
of Nordau's paradigms of health as harmony with the natural
world on the one hand, and sickness as a selfish craving for the
artificial stimuli of contemporary society on the other, is not
surprising.[46] According to Nordau, it is the constitutional
weakness 'among those whose nervous life is more or less
diseased, namely, among hysterical, neurasthenic, and degenerate subjects, and every kind of lunatic' which renders them so

[46] Gissing read Max Nordau's *Degeneration* in March 1895, a month after its
publication in England. See Pierre Coustillas (ed.), *London and the Life of
Literature in Late Victorian England: The Diary of George Gissing, Novelist*
(Brighton: Harvester Press, 1978), p. 365.

susceptible to sense impressions that their lives are irremediably governed by what he calls 'organic emotion'.[47] Such impressionability entails a restlessness and dislocation which impede the natural concordance with external reality that is generally considered to be the *sine qua non* of physical, mental, and moral well-being. The belief that vital forces traversed between organism and environment had been astonishingly tenacious, re-emerging at different times in ever more scientifically sophisticated forms. Dowse now concurred with the prominent physician William Withey Gull in the proposition that the organic and inorganic worlds are built of the same elements. 'Life' or 'vitality', they were persuaded, should be understood as a refined form of the same energy that exists in the inorganic world. Conceptualized thus, Gull had argued, the 'organization of our bodies in relation to the earth we inhabit' is merely 'the expression of the highest correlation of these external conditions'.[48] As developments in the understanding of electrical power and the nervous system brought these two models of energy into close scientific proximity, it made sense that the healthy body required a natural balance of the positive and negative charges which, it was believed, flowed through the natural world. The sensitive individual was, therefore, profoundly affected by the natural electrical changes in the atmosphere and his or her nervous system easily thrown out of balance by man-made stimulations.[49] In novels, environment is often portrayed as the hostile or benign medium that will foster or suppress latent morbid or healthy traits and tendencies. Houses and location are of paramount importance in *The Whirlpool*, in defining and determining the health or sickness of those individuals who inhabit them. The Mortons's house, Greystone, is a country-town idyll, a haven of domestic tranquillity and untrammelled good sense, which is seamlessly interwoven with the sentimental idealist view of life the Mortons themselves present. Similarly, the elegant London apartments are consistent with the traffic and intrigue of *demi-monde*

---

[47] *Degeneration*, p. 476.
[48] William Withey Gull, Harveian oration at the Royal College of Physicians (1870). Cited by Dowse in *On Brain and Nerve Exhaustion*, p. 16.
[49] See John S. and Robin M. Haller, *The Physician and Sexuality in Victorian America* (Chicago: University of Illinois Press, 1974), p. 12.

transience, as are suburban Pinner and Gunnersbury with Alma's oscillations between frenzied involvement and marginal gentility.[50]

From his first acquaintance with her, Rolfe had observed what he took to be the 'natural' and 'inevitable' process by which Alma 'absorbed the vulgarity of her atmosphere' (41). Each of Alma's moves, and her brief sojourns in Europe, are directly related to the fluctuations in her state of health. It is during the early years of their married life in rural Wales that Alma's antipathies towards their unadorned self-sufficiency manifest themselves in fainting fits and attacks of hysteria. While Rolfe is invigorated by the bucolic life, he recognizes that, for his wife, 'the solitude was telling upon her nerves' (161). When she suffers what can only be construed as a miscarriage, her 'illness' is implicitly, but unmistakably, attributed to a self-generated dread of enforced domesticity, made worse by envy of her husband's and Mrs Abbott's unconstrained freedom. Working herself into a frenzy, the reluctant mother contrives an act of deliberate recklessness. Alma's perilous lone drive in the dogcart to overtake the unsuspecting pair on their walk prompts Rolfe to ponder the morbid implications of his wife's erratic behaviour. As her illness takes its course, he is alarmed by the unnaturalness of Alma's unconcealed relief at having been spared any encumbrance to her present freedom. That which 'some women would have wept over' came as a 'blessing' to his wife, even bringing 'joy into her eyes' (162). From a moral standpoint, however, he has no grounds to condemn Alma for not desiring her own child when he himself had long pontificated on the evils of bringing unwanted children into the world.[51] But, although there are no rational arguments for the different natures of husband and wife here, Alma's feminine instincts are constantly invoked in terms of vital energies innately antithetical to those which inspire her husband. Their incompatibility in this regard is reminiscent of Hardy's Eustacia

[50] These migrations were also, of course, a reality of nineteenth-century middle-class life. Few readers of Victorian (auto)biography can have failed to be struck by the frequency with which people moved around from place to place, repeatedly taking properties in the pursuit of, variously: health, rest, tranquillity; or society, activity, culture.

[51] See *The Whirlpool*, pp. 13, 20, and 184.

Vye and Clym Yeobright, whose nerve forces were distinctly
charged by the separate worlds of a dream of Parisian elegance
and the rustic simplicity of Egdon Heath.[52]

Along with environment, the other crucial factor in nervous
degeneration was, of course, heredity. In *The Whirlpool*, as in
Jude the Obscure, ancestry is the dead hand which commits its
unfortunate legatees to inevitable dissolution. When Rolfe's
suspicions are aroused by Alma's fluctuations between excessive
expenditure of energy and nervous prostration, he begins to
look for clues in her family history. After the birth of Hughie,
he had taken to 'reading and musing much on questions of
heredity' (136) to seek explanations for his wife's seeming lack
of interest in the nurturing necessities of motherhood. Great
significance is laid upon the discovery that Alma's mother had
collapsed and died of a brain haemorrhage caused by, it was
said, her over-excitement after a visit to the theatre. Her father,
as Rolfe already knows, committed suicide on account of his
business failure—an act which, in the 1890s, was considered
psychologically and morally inseparable from the morbid loss
of will-power signalling encroaching insanity. Gissing's interpretation is in tune with degenerationist discourse and the
significant role it had lately assumed in neurological case study.
If, as was claimed, recklessness is one of the unquestionable
precipitants of neurasthenia in those individuals who have
inherited an already depleted nerve force, intelligence of the
medical history of our forebears must act as a rule of thumb to
indicate an absolute requirement to conserve energy by living a
life of quiet moderation. Rolfe himself acts according to a model
of conservation and self-preservation, whilst Alma displays the
characteristic self-delusion of the neurasthenic, adding to her
resource debit by obsessively craving the admiration of friends
for her energy and determination.[53]

---

[52] Thomas Hardy, *The Return of the Native* (1878). On 15 September 1895,
Gissing writes in his diary of a visit to Thomas Hardy in Dorchester during which
they walked 'to the edge of "Egdon Heath". Hardy talking a little about his new
book which is to be called "Jude the Obscure" '. See Pierre Coustillas, *London and
the Life of Literature*, p. 387.

[53] Dowse had gloomily forecast that 'the *very effort* to will annihilates will-
power. So with the neurasthenic, [. . .] consciousness of a desire to will inhibits the
power to will'. *On Brain and Nerve Exhaustion*, p. 30, emphasis in original.

Alma Rolfe, like so many fictional women of her time who sought a measure of independence and self-fulfilment, is in a vortex, suspended between depressive illness ensuing from domestic boredom and isolation and nervous collapse due to her unceasing participation in the whirl and fury of modern life. Yet, in her own words, she is conscious of being 'on the outer edge of the whirlpool'. Marriage conferred a respectability on her which she exploits as the means of allowing herself 'more freedom of movement than was permissible to single young women' (188). Gissing's readiness to pathologize her restless commuting between the margins of respectable suburbia and the hub of social activity masks more rational explanations for her agitation or her drained and nerveless pallor. For instance, in the immediate aftermath of Alma's musical debut she suffers a complete nervous collapse not on account of the physical and mental exertion of the concert itself but of shock upon subsequently learning of Hugh Carnaby's sudden disappearance following the murder of Cyrus Redgrave. Indeed, Alma is in no doubt that her violent nervous reaction was not precipitated by the strains of concert performance. On the contrary, 'the one marvellous thing' about it, she recalls, 'was her absolute conquest of nervousness' (315), her glorious delight in the 'mastery of her instrument' and her consciousness of playing 'without effort, and could have played for hours without weariness' (313). But yet Rolfe later tells Carnaby that she 'has made herself ill' with a nervous breakdown brought on by the 'concert, and the frenzy that went before it' (319–20). Uncomfortable inconsistencies are simply ironed out as the narrative of Alma's decline goes hand in hand with her excursions into the public sphere. From the 'severe headache [which] had left behind it some nervous disorder, not to be shaken off by any effort' (263–4), to the hysterical outburst which left Rolfe recalling Bennet Frothingham's suicide (446), Alma's deteriorating health is causally related by Gissing to a reckless, mismanaged, inappropriate lifestyle. Over-excitement and over-stimulation take their toll upon the nerves and the more Alma seeks rational explanation for her fears and suspicions, the more irrational her actions are made to seem in the eyes of observers and commentators.

Moreover, the registration of inherited susceptibilities shows similar inconsistencies. Whilst at pains to stress Alma's hardly propitious mental and physiological inheritance, the narrator attributes her healthier moments to parental sources which are not borne out by their medical history:

Alma lay down with a contented sigh, and was soon asleep, thanks to the health she still enjoyed. Her excitability was of the imagination rather than of the blood, and the cool, lymphatic flow, characteristically feminine, which mingled with the sanguine humour, traceable perhaps to a paternal source, spared her many an hour of wakefulness, as it guarded her against much graver peril.   (228)

When even the mention of Bennet Frothingham's name is enough to cast a terrible shadow over Alma's social and constitutional credentials, it seems incongruous to attribute the 'health she still enjoyed' to the 'sanguine humour, traceable perhaps to a paternal source'. Equally, if it was from her mother that she inherited her excitability of the imagination- the mother who 'died suddenly, after an evening at the theatre, where, as usual, she had excited herself beyond measure' (136)—it is difficult to know what to make of the description of the 'cool, lymphatic flow' which coursed through Alma's veins as 'characteristically feminine' (228). These and other incongruities testify to the precariousness of attempting to map rigid medical categories or aetiological rules onto the fugitive workings of human behaviour. Even the most assured theoretical pronouncements on the interrelation of heredity, habitat, and human health begin to disperse in the whirlpool of experience. As if acknowledging this process of dissolution, Gissing has Rolfe abandon a position of confident supremacy with regard to his own ideas when experience weakens his resolve, but then, unlike with Alma, assigns altruistic rather than egotistic motives for his vacillation.

Early in the novel, Rolfe's remedy for the parlous state of the national health, with 'some of us sunk in barbarism, some coddling themselves in over-refinement' (14), lies unequivocally in the promotion of male vigour and moral fibre in order to sustain England's military might. By the end he is much less certain about the virtues of imperialism and, in the matter of his son Hughie's education, errs on the side of the very 'softness and sweetness of civilisation' (449) he had earlier deplored. The clamorous campaign to 'look to our physique, and make ourselves ready' is ridiculed by Rolfe along with the present trend for turning games into battles on the fields of sport, and it is with a nervous ambivalence on his part that he mediates his militaristic fervour to his son through the reading of Kipling's 'Barrack-Room Ballads'. It is often argued that Rolfe's doubts and equivocation are consistent with an unmanly indecisiveness which parallels Gissing's own cramped sense of existing in a void between a culture of progress and repressive gentility, where 'energetic individualism' seems to be as utterly futile as entrenched traditionalism.[54] Having read *Degeneration*, Gissing must have been conscious of Nordau's jaundiced interpretation of abject pessimism in the contemporary novel. According to Nordau, this negative quality was the unmistakable mark of degeneracy which linked writer and his creation together in a downward spiral of psychic and somatic enervation. Ambivalence, it might be argued, works to resist dissolution by avoiding the perils both of exhaustion through too much expenditure of energy and atrophy through too little. But when, in the final chapter, Rolfe's self-confessed inability to 'make up his mind on any subject of thought' spreads over into an anxiety that his 'waverings and doubtings' (452) may have irremediably affected Hughie, the gentle, contemplative way of life he has adopted for his son's sake seems as potentially injurious as the frenzied vortex it was meant to replace. If New Woman and New Man are equally destined to dissolution, who are to be the representatives of healthy regeneration?

Despite Gissing's leaving of Harvey Rolfe in the expansive bosom of the Mortons, optimistic notions of healthy regeneration in this novel, as in Hardy, are either conspicuously absent or overshadowed with negative images of female sexuality. With the exception of Mrs Morton and, to a lesser extent, Mrs Abbott, *The Whirlpool* is scathing in its depictions of the female characters. In the same spirit that doctors and social commentators seized upon mental difference between men and women to link the incidence of female nervous disease to their acts of emancipation, Gissing constructed a world of female experience that

[54] For example, John Sloan, *George Gissing: The Cultural Challenge* (London: Macmillan, 1989). See also David Grylls, *The Paradox of Gissing* (London: Allen and Unwin, 1986).

was the pathological antithesis of a male vision of utopia. Whether that world mirrors the reality of nervous degeneration or the selfish indulgence of a fashionable fad, to Gissing's mind, its proprietors were women. Alma's decline into neurasthenic symptoms of fatigue, insomnia, irritability, and depression leading finally to her overdose of opium might be taken straight from Dowse's diagnosis of brain and nerve consumption as the direct consequence of the reckless expenditure of energy from an already deficient reserve. At the same time, the text alludes disparagingly to her 'fashionable disorder of the nerves' (305), adopted for its social cachet or, more calculatedly, for the avoidance of domestic duties. She is vilified by Hugh Carnaby for her selfishness in 'running at large about London, giving concerts, making herself ill and ugly, whilst her little son was left to a governess and servants' (279). Nor is she the only woman whose malady is derided on account of its suspected self-indulgence. Mrs Leach, whose solicitor husband 'had no function in life but to toil without pause for the support of his family in genteel leisure' (187) was free to suffer 'from some obscure affection of the nerves, which throughout the whole of her married life had disabled her from paying any continuous regard to domestic affairs' and her debility had 'now reached such a point that the unfortunate lady could do nothing but collapse in chairs and loll on sofas' (186). If Mrs Leach's nervousness is a mark of respectability, Mrs Strangeways's neuralgic pains strongly suggest the opposite. Her dismissive reply to Alma's enquiry after her health that 'my neuralgic something or other' is 'the price one pays for civilisation' (264–5) conceals more sinister connotations of the increased disease susceptibility associated with urban circulation. Her 'over-scented, over-heated boudoir' turned Alma's thoughts to 'the things unspeakable which always seemed to her to be lurking in the shadowed corners of Mrs Strangeways' house' (164). With 'strange' ways carrying connotations of aberrance and sexual transgression, this *demi-monde* hostess with her 'pallid, hollow-eyed look of illness' is the contagious link in the chain of physical as well as moral contamination.

Mrs Abbott is unusual in transforming, in Harvey Rolfe's eyes at least, from a small-minded, 'slightly peevish', and cross woman, whom Rolfe more than half believes might have driven her husband to his untimely death, into one whom the years had rendered more compliant. Experience, he opined, had made her 'a better woman' and she is 'rewarded', finally, by a suitable marriage and the concomitant release from an irksome career. The only model of womanhood which would have met, for example, with Herbert Spencer's approval is that of Mrs Morton, whose domestic idyll is manifestly a sentimental idealization. As a picture of maternal perfection and the guarantee of future vigour, Mrs Morton's successful breeding is clearly meant to be set against Alma's quivering inadequacy. We are told that, unlike Alma, who seeks self-fulfilment outside the home not within it, and who gives birth to 'a lamentable little mortal with a voice scarcely louder than a kitten's' (387) who dies at only two weeks old, Mrs Morton entertained no 'conflict with motherhood. Her breasts were the fountain of life; her babies clung to them, and grew large of limb. . . . She would have felt it an impossible thing to abandon her children to the care of servants' (324) while she went into society. But if the negative images are embodiments of the specific anxieties besetting the age, the portrait of the dutiful Mrs Morton is self-confessedly a dream 'after the old fashion' (324), a nostalgic reinvention of the angel in the house.

In the case of Alma Rolfe, the pace of modern life exhausted and finally overwhelmed a woman whose ability to withstand stress and strain was already much diminished by her having inherited a constitution which fails under duress. Her father, Bennet Frothingham, had been a classic case of the type of businessman whom doctors like Dowse were attending all too frequently in recent years; resolute men, men 'of great capacity and business powers', but who launch out too far in the pursuit of capital gain until their empires crumble and they are 'crushed by opposing forces'.[55] In themselves, the pathogenic consequences of such imprudent expansion were not unexpected, and had indeed been recognized at least since George Cheyne warned of the health costs of prosperity and progress in his study *The English Malady* of 1733. But what brought the added dimension of powerlessness to the clinical picture of breakdown in the 1890s was the belief in the stranglehold of cumulative

[55] *On Brain and Nerve Exhaustion*, p. 27.

degeneracy, a process whereby the experiences of one generation are never erased, but live on in the biological 'memory' of the next.

While those doctors who were prepared to add neurasthenia to their diagnostic canon were in agreement about inherited nervous depletion as a fact of progressive degeneration, not all were persuaded that modern urban life was responsible for the emergence of a new disease. Clifford Allbutt, for example, disputed this and other aetiological claims, and warned, in an article in the *Contemporary Review*, that new names do not make new diseases but merely enable the 'fashionable fad of the day' to bestow itself with scientific verification.[56] Allbutt, a prominent physician known to Thomas Hardy through their membership of The Savile Club, was one of only a few medical men who were prepared to admit that the preoccupation with speculative and often prejudiced theories of causation hindered the search for more accurate paradigms for mind/body boundaries and, therefore, more effective conceptions of physical and mental disease.[57] He rejected, for instance, the notion that intellectual intensity was ever a cause of nervous collapse, and flew in the face of many of his colleagues in pointing to the men and, importantly, women also, whose lives had been only enriched and enhanced by the pursuit of high academic goals. Critics of the *fin de siècle* have cited 'Nervous Diseases and Modern Life' to strengthen the causal connection between social change and female neurosis.[58] But the whole point of Allbutt's article is to challenge the belief that the whirlpool of modern life is, of itself, injurious to health. When we hear, he argues, and every day see 'neurotics, neurasthenics, hysterics, and the like' and 'every

[56] T. Clifford Allbutt, 'Nervous Diseases and Modern Life', *Contemporary Review*, 67 (1895), 210–31 (p. 217).

[57] It is recorded in *The Life of Thomas Hardy* that in May 1891 Hardy 'was much impressed by a visit paid with his friend Dr (later Sir) T. Clifford Allbutt, then a Commissioner in Lunacy, to a large private lunatic asylum' (p. 236). Two years later he participated in 'a scientific evening at the *conversazione* of the Royal Society, where I talked on the exhibits to Sir R. Quain, Dr. Clifford Allbutt, Humphry Ward, Bosworth Smith, Sir J. Crichton-Browne, F. and G. Macmillan, Ray Lankester, and others, without (I flatter myself) betraying excessive ignorance in respect of the points in the show' (p. 254). Hardy continued to meet Allbutt and Crichton-Browne at the dinners and lectures of the Medico-Psychological Society.

[58] Elaine Showalter in *Sexual Anarchy*, p. 40 and William Greenslade in *Degeneration, Culture and the Novel*, pp. 137–8.

large city filled with nerve-specialists, and their chambers with patients'; with 'hospitals, baths, electric-machines, and massages multiplying daily for their use; nerve-tonics sold behind every counter, and health-resorts advertised for their solace and restoration' the *apparent* increase in 'neurotic traffic' is due simply to the increase in comparatively 'well, rich and idle people', to fashionable physicians only too ready to pander to their delusions, and to the incitement of alarm by a mischievous media.[59]

It could be objected that Allbutt's fervent denial of the existence of global decline and his overturning of the popular picture of a present generation of urban neurotics set much of his work in contradistinction to Hardy's more pessimistic view of the world. But what is particularly interesting about his writing in relation to that of Hardy in the 1890s is a shared understanding that nervous disease and environment were much more complexly related than the phrase 'modern life stress' seemed to allow. It is this sense of complexity that distinguishes Hardy's representation of neurasthenia from Gissing's. Sue Bridehead's collapse is not so much brought on by foolish recklessness or over-exertion, as by merely attempting to deal with the world as it is. Nervous degeneration was, for Hardy, an inevitable consequence of what he saw as an ever-widening gap between material (urban and technological) and human (spiritual and emotional) progress. It was as if the material world of the late nineteenth century demanded a level of toughness and stamina for which the more highly developed, cerebral individuals among humankind were not fitted. The depressing inference seemed to be a falling off in the human capacity to keep pace with its own inventions and its own intellectual enlightenment. In 1888 Hardy had expressed his disquiet thus:

A woeful fact—that the human race is too extremely developed for its corporeal conditions, the nerves being evolved to an activity abnormal in such an environment. Even the higher animals are in excess in this respect. It may be questioned if Nature, or what we call Nature, so far back as when she crossed the line from invertebrates to vertebrates, did not exceed her mission. This planet does not supply the materials for happiness to higher existences.[60]

---

[59] 'Nervous Diseases and Modern Life', p. 217.
[60] *The Life of Thomas Hardy*, p. 218.

REFINEMENT AND REVERSION IN *JUDE THE OBSCURE*

In the 1912 postscript to the Preface to the first edition of *Jude*, Hardy responded in a non-committal way to the German reviewer who characterized Sue Bridehead as 'the slight, pale "bachelor" girl—the intellectualized, emancipated bundle of nerves that modern conditions were producing, mainly in cities as yet' (xxxviii). On this, and previous occasions, his refusal to be drawn on the subject of the New Woman merely indicates that his book has broader concerns than just that of using nervous collapse as a moral judgement on a certain type of woman. The representation of Sue Bridehead draws unmistakably upon current beliefs and attitudes concerning gender variation within the tortuous equation of biological determinism and modern trends. But it is also fair to argue, as Penny Boumelha has done, that Hardy's heroine is not 'representative' of a movement or group.[61] Rather, she is created more for the purposes of exploring the ideological currents which sweep her along than simply to illustrate their unpalatable features.

Hardy's pessimistic view that human faculties had somehow become out of step with the developmental laws of nature was applied to both sexes equally. 'We [human beings]', he wrote in 1883, 'have reached a degree of intelligence which Nature never contemplated when framing her laws, and for which she consequently has provided no adequate satisfactions'.[62] Later he compounded this disjunction with the wry observation quoted above that the nervous system had evolved to a level of sensitivity which had outgrown the 'corporeal conditions' to which it was still functionally bound. In the novel, Hardy puts the very same thought into the mind of the intelligently imaginative Sue, who is haunted by the idea that 'at the framing of the terrestrial conditions there seemed never to have been contemplated such a development of emotional perceptiveness among the creatures subject to those conditions as that reached by thinking and educated humanity' (361). Hardy's much-quoted phrase, the 'deadly war waged between flesh and spirit', points ominously

---

[61] Penny Boumelha, *Thomas Hardy and Women: Sexual Ideology and Narrative Form* (Brighton: Harvester Press, 1982), p. 137.
[62] *The Life of Thomas Hardy*, p. 163.

to what he saw as, in evolutionary terms, an unprecedented clash of interests between the higher cerebral and neural functions unique to humankind and the fleshly instincts which belonged to Darwin's 'past and lower state of civilisation'.[63] The struggle to come to terms with a sexuality which does not compromise high-minded principles or aspirations is one which, for different reasons, possesses both Sue and Jude. Although this is to over-simplify that struggle, their failure to settle the antagonism is perhaps a testimony to the error of perceiving flesh and spirit as mutually exclusive choices in a conflict which must be decided.

If the reconciliation of opposing forces is problematic for both protagonists, it is Sue whose nerves give way under the strain. For Jude, the desires of the flesh are, if not the fault of women, the 'gins and springes' which the 'system of things' strews in the path 'to noose and hold back those who want to progress' (228). Reflecting as to his fitness to be a man of the church, he accepts somewhat resignedly that, 'taken all round, he was a man of too many passions to make a good clergyman; the utmost he could hope for was that in a life of constant internal warfare between flesh and spirit the former might not always be victorious' (201). For Sue, on the other hand, such a compromise is not so easily negotiated since female sexuality had no tradition of expression other than through the channels of marriage and maternity. Her reluctance to accept such a narrow prescription and her corresponding desire for new freedoms are the 'unnatural' traits which she shares with the New Woman, and the same traits which persuaded some critics that her creator intended her as a representative type.[64] But if Sue is pathologized by Jude for being unnatural as a woman, the question of whether she is sick because she is a woman and, by long inurement of nature, deemed physiologically and emotionally unequal to the tasks she now sets herself, is rooted in the text's sexual political self-consciousness. The probability of a mental difference between men and women strikes Jude early in his acquaintance with Sue when he remarks on a disposition which Maudsley and others had identified as being characteristically

---

[63] Charles Darwin, *The Descent of Man*, p. 564.
[64] Postscript, Preface to the 1st edn., p. xxxviii.

female. In the passage from *The Physiology of Mind* quoted earlier, the authoritative voice of essentialist mentality defined 'a subjective class marked by the tendency to feel intensely rather than to see clearly', a class of mind lower in the scale of evolution which owes more to 'self-feeling' than to ratiocination.[65] It is not merely on account of his callowness that Sue appears to Jude as 'a revelation of woman' in so far as 'everything she did seemed to have its source in feeling' (104). The recognition of mental difference which at first delights, but later exasperates, Jude is in line with contemporary scientific attempts to explain female impressionability, intuition, and feeling as rooted in the law of nature. Jude's attempt to understand and interpret Sue is thwarted by contradictions in that very science which linked women's nervous disease both to their arrested development and a nervous sensitivity that had become over-refined.

But Jude's perceptions are themselves shown to be distorted and erroneous. Hardy's curiosity about the psychology of perception and of perceptual error is evidenced in his notebooks where he copied passages from Maudsley's *Natural Causes and Supernatural Seemings* during the period 1888–90.[66] As Patricia Gallivan has shown, 'Jude moves through what Maudsley calls a "process of progressive disillusioning", a correction of error in "seeing and believing" '.[67] The ' "coming to know" of the novel form' is Jude's increasing realization that his perceptual powers betrayed him and that his dreams were mere delusions. The problem of accurate or erroneous interpretation of the meaning of things is one which is not Jude's alone, but is shared by the narrator, by the reader, and is persistently present throughout the text as a reminder of what Hardy understood to be the fallibility of all human endeavour in the face of the implacable laws of science. However, within that general model, individual failure is shown to elicit significantly different kinds of response from hero and heroine.

---

[65] *The Physiology of Mind*, p. 377.

[66] Henry Maudsley, *Natural Causes and Supernatural Seemings* (London: Kegan Paul, Trench, 1886). For a differently inflected reading of theories of perception in Hardy's writing, see J. B. Bullen, *The Expressive Eye: Fiction and Perception in the Work of Thomas Hardy* (Oxford: Clarendon Press, 1986).

[67] Patricia Gallivan, 'Science and Art in *Jude the Obscure*', in Anne Smith (ed.), *The Novels of Thomas Hardy* (London: Vision Press, 1979), pp. 126–44 (p. 133).

There is a point, shortly after the deaths of the children, where Jude and Sue diverge into the gendered patterns of mental functioning laid down by evolutionary biologists and psychiatrists. Jude reasons his way out of the pit of despair by re-proportioning the events to which Sue attaches huge moral and religious significance into the purposeless reality of 'man and senseless circumstance' (361). It would, of course, be foolish to deny the causal connection between the tragedy that befalls the family and Sue's subsequent breakdown. My point is that, in depicting Sue's collapse, Hardy, no less than Gissing, assimilates the rhetoric of inferior female organization and of mental difference, but, unlike Gissing, does not simply reproduce it as though it were fact. Hardy's interest is in the psychosexual rather than the merely sexual aspects of difference. His exposition of nervous disintegration reveals, therefore, a much more complex interaction of inherited and acquired attributes than the picture of mental incapacity and exhausted resources painted in some late-nineteenth-century texts would suggest. It is true that Sue's nervous disintegration takes the form of a reversal to prescribed norms of womanhood. But this capitulation on Sue's part is no concession to science of the evolutionary argument against emancipation. Indeed, Sue's belief that the catastrophe is a punishment for her aberrant notions is presented, unequivocally, as a sign of her advancing illness. Hardy's purpose is to explore a multiplicity of interrelated factors, cultural as well as psychological and physiological, in bringing about Sue's reversal.

Accordingly, Sue's peculiarly individual psychosexual identity is no sooner stated than thrown open to challenge. Sue is eager to tell Jude that she is different from other women, that her 'life has been entirely shaped by what people call a peculiarity in me' (152). But the narrator is puzzled as to whether Sue behaves as she does because she is a woman or because she just happens to be a perverse individual. That '[w]omen were different from men' in their attitudes to relationships is offered at first as sufficient explanation of Sue's incomprehensible thoughtlessness in asking Jude to give her away in marriage to Phillotson, but is then immediately reconsidered:

Was it that they were, instead of more sensitive, *as reputed*, more callous, and less romantic; or were they more heroic? Or was Sue simply so perverse that she wilfully gave herself and him pain for the odd and mournful luxury of practising long-suffering in her own person, and of being touched with tender pity for him at having made him practise it? He could perceive that her face was nervously set, and when they reached the trying ordeal of Jude giving her to Phillotson she could hardly command herself; . . . Possibly she would go on inflicting such pains again and again, and grieving for the sufferer again and again, in all her colossal inconsistency. . . . Could it be that Sue had acted with such unusual foolishness as to plunge into she knew not what for the sake of asserting her independence of him, of retaliating on him for his secrecy? Perhaps Sue was thus venturesome with men because she was childishly ignorant of that side of their natures which wore out women's hearts and lives. (181–2, my emphasis)

Essentialist views of emotional, intellectual, and behavioural traits are not difficult to find in this text. But even in their expression they come up against the problem of explaining female exceptionality within a discourse of natural subordination. For this reason, they cannot be taken at face value. As the passage shows, such views are most often expressed not in the form of statements but as questions proceeding from bewilderment. In fact, Jude is later driven, upon Sue's decision to return to Phillotson following the deaths of the children, to put again the very questions which perplex the narrator. 'What I can't understand in you', he agonizes, 'is your extraordinary blindness now to your old logic. Is it peculiar to you, or is it common to Woman? Is a woman a thinking unit at all, or a fraction always wanting its integer?' (370). Hardy makes essential difference between the sexes a function of Jude's misunderstanding. In his desperation to explain Sue's attitudes and behaviour, he turns to conventional wisdoms which are in line with what evolutionist medicine identified as an inherently female class of mind. Of course Hardy excludes Sue from such an essentialist category but, in so doing, he binds her to a pathology of nervous disintegration allied to the strain of being different.

Sue's self-proclaimed difference from other women is repeatedly stressed both directly and suggestively, as is the case when her absence from the long line of 'tender feminine faces' in the students' dormitory implies her exclusion from its ideology of passive submission. At first, she is at pains to impress Jude with her radical notions, shocking him by questioning the authority of chronology and of attribution in the Epistles and Gospels (157). Far from being merely capricious, her iconoclasm raises the huge question of the arbitrariness of meaning when order is imposed on to a purposeless void. Neither Phillotson nor Jude can respond to her scepticism about the authenticity of the artefacts in an exhibition of Christ's Jerusalem in anything other than a somewhat patronizing recognition of her 'cleverness' for a woman. And yet, unwilling to pursue the point in the manner of a more committed and outspoken New Woman, Sue quickly withdraws, self-consciously announcing 'I hate to be what is called a clever girl—there are too many of that sort now!' (109). If Sue has none of the 'messianic sense of purpose which distinguishes her contemporaries' in the works of George Egerton or Grant Allen, her eagerness to present herself as an individual with an originality of mind was sufficient to impress the writer of *Keynotes*.[68] Originality, however, was a faculty little admired in women since it stood dangerously at variance with the more acceptable feminine qualities of reactivity and compliance.

The dilemma as to whether Sue's ideas and behaviour showed signs of an extraordinary refinement of the senses or an aberrant psychology is somewhat hastily resolved by linking the two together so that her intelligence is presented as inseparable from 'the perverseness that was part of her' (138). If the conjunction of intelligence and perversity was a necessary requisite for exceptionality it was also, and most particularly for women, potentially injurious. In Sue's case it leaves her suspended in a void between a visionary, though inchoate, sense of new freedoms and the perpetually frustrated desire to dissociate herself from enslavement to prescribed forms of social and sexual duty. When she tells Jude about her former friendship with the undergraduate who died, she expresses her exceptionality in terms of being free of the sexual self-objectification that 'most women *are taught* to feel' (152, my emphasis) by men and their books. Most contemporary reviewers saw Sue's exceptionality as essentially sick, her perversity as the registrations of 'disease in an

---

[68] Penny Boumelha, *Thomas Hardy and Women*, p. 137. For a discussion of the similarities between Hardy's Sue and George Egerton's heroine in 'A Cross Line', see Gail Cunningham, *The New Woman and the Victorian Novel*, pp. 105–6.

incurably morbid organism'.[69] R. Y. Tyrell puts her intellectual curiosity down to a 'fantastic green-sickness' and her frantic need to analyse relationships down to her 'warped and neurotic nature'.[70] Edmund Gosse, perhaps momentarily forgetful that Jude and Sue descend from the same doomed family, describes Sue alone as a 'maimed "degenerate" ' and 'a strange and unwelcome product of exhaustion'.[71] Hardy had defended his heroine's 'abnormalism', describing it as consisting in 'disproportion, not in inversion'. Protesting against critical accusations of perversion and depravity in Sue's nature, however, he quantifies her womanliness as depletion of desire, whereby her 'sexual instinct' is 'healthy as far so it goes, but unusually weak and fastidious', and excess of nervous sensibilities, which 'remain painfully alert . . . as they do in nature with such women'.[72] In this way, he inscribes her singularity in terms of the general imbalance he claimed to observe between refined sensitivities and primitive instinct in the modern world.

The link between originality of mind and nervous instability had a long history. Henry Maudsley had brought much of his earlier work on diseased consciousness into the era of degeneration panic when he designated a pathological category for the mind that dared to be different and to 'rebel against the established rule'.[73] The force of originality needed to make a stand against the custom and routine of one's allotted medium is a property only of the unstable brain, he averred. And Hardy noted how this type was most frequently to be found in individuals of 'a distinct neurotic strain—sometimes a strain of madness—in their families'.[74] Such an unhappy conjunction is the 'transcendent irony of fate' since it bound the pioneering spirit to a finite and diminishing supply of nervous energy. Having discharged itself in striving for 'a high moral ideal' or of 'new surroundings, of an evolutionary or revolutional character',

[69] R. Y. Tyrell, *Fortnightly Review* (June 1896), cited in *Thomas Hardy: The Critical Heritage*, ed. by R. G. Cox (London: Routledge and Kegan Paul, 1970), p. 295.

[70] *The Critical Heritage*, p. 295.

[71] Edmund Gosse, *Cosmopolis* (January 1896), cited in *The Critical Heritage*, pp. 268–9.

[72] *The Life of Thomas Hardy*, p. 272.   [73] *Natural Causes*, p. 208.

[74] See *The Literary Notebooks of Thomas Hardy*, ed. by Lennart A. Björk, 2 vols. (London: Macmillan, 1985), i, pp. 198–201 (p. 198).

that energy is soon exhausted.[75] Maudsley's vicious circle of inevitable disintegration was grist to the mill of the pessimist. Perhaps this is why his evermore elusory scientism appealed to Hardy as he worked to create a heroine whose peculiar notions are the mark of her originality but, at the same time, signal her unfitness, because of her defective ancestry, to survive the vicissitudes that her own disruptive energies had stirred into action.

When Sue's nerves give way, her breakdown, unlike Jude's disillusioning and demise, has little to do with the general 'FAILURE of THINGS to be what they are meant to be'.[76] Rather, it takes a much more specific form of nervous and psychological degeneration. Sue's crisis precipitates a stage-by-stage return to the old duties and conventions which her healthier mind had been so resolute against. It is a paradox of her condition that her reversion to a quivering, self-sacrificial domestic angel is at once a symptom of her disease and a sign of reintegration into a prescribed norm within a stable sexual hierarchy. Corresponding in principle to Maudsley's exposition of the 'transcendent irony of fate—that the complete accomplishment of disillusion shall be the close of development and the beginning of degeneration', Sue's nervous collapse is precipitated by the deaths of the children and marks the demise of the degenerative line.[77] For Hardy's heroine, the 'close of development' and the 'beginning of degeneration' are both familial and personal turning-points. Unhinged by this crisis, Sue suffers what Maudsley saw as a 'reversion to the old belief of savages'.[78] Her alarm that 'I am getting as superstitious as a savage' is confirmation of her own retreat from participation in present 'thinking and educated humanity' but it is also an emerging symptom of immutable atavistic continuity.

Jude's tragedy lies in his realization both of his own failure and of the incompatibility of a pioneering modernity and an

[75] Maudsley, *Natural Causes*, p. 209. The phrase 'a high moral ideal' appears in Hardy's transcription though not in Maudsley's text. See *The Literary Notebooks*, i, p. 198.

[76] *The Life of Thomas Hardy*, p. 124, emphasis in original.

[77] *Natural Causes*, p. 367.

[78] Patricia Gallivan identifies Sue's regression into 'guilt and fear and orthodoxy' precisely in these Maudsleyan terms. See 'Science and Art in *Jude the Obscure*', p. 133. The Maudsley quotation is from *Natural Causes*, p. 161.

obdurate world. Even in the troughs of his misery and acceler-
ating disease he manages to reflect with philosophical detachment that the problem had always been that '[o]ur ideas were
fifty years too soon to be any good to us' (422–3). Sue, on the
other hand, turns away from the clear light of intellect to the
point where Jude fears she may have lost her reason. Her reversion attests once more to the dynamic contradiction between
progressive refinement and the inescapable burden of a tainted
inheritance. Both protagonists have their origins in the same
weak stock with its history of marital breakdown, illness,
suicide, and insanity. From childhood it had been impressed
upon them equally that they 'belonged to an odd and peculiar
family—the wrong breed for marriage' (174). 'There's sommat
in our blood', Aunt Drusilla had divined, in an unwitting allusion to Weismann's immutable germ-plasm, 'that won't take
kindly to the notion of being bound to do what we do readily
enough if not bound' (70). In a letter to a friend, Hardy had
confided that his concerns in the novel were not so much with
the marriage question in general, as was too often assumed, as
with a very particular instance of 'the tragic issues of two bad
marriages, owing in the main to a doom or curse of hereditary
temperament peculiar to the family of the parties'.[79] With
resources already depleted by an adverse genealogy, Sue's capacity for exercising volitional control over her thoughts and
actions begins to fail and she surrenders, body and mind, to the
tyrannical government of the nerves. That point where health
turns to disease is marked metaphorically as a turning from
light to darkness, from enlightenment to a primitive past, and is
encapsulated in Jude's rueful observation that Sue 'was once a
woman whose intellect was to mine like a star to a benzoline
lamp' but which is now broken by affliction and 'veered round
to darkness' (422).

Once out of reach of the controlling influence of the will, the
disordered mind can no longer progress but resorts instead,
according to Maudsley, to the 'active revival or recrudescence of
a surviving superstition'.[80] It is not insignificant that Sue's
nervous breakdown takes the form of a mortification of the

---

[79] *The Life of Thomas Hardy*, p. 271.
[80] *Natural Causes*, p. 161.

flesh, a process which links physiological degeneration and religious mania, itself diagnosed as hysterical neurosis by those medical scientists for whom religion and 'surviving superstition' were one and the same. By implicitly making this connection, Hardy presents diminution of the will as at once a necessary requirement and a sign of neurological disease. In the religious context it is a prerequisite of the supplicant's humility whilst, in the neurological, it marks the abandonment of the rational and civilized self to the erratic and unpredictable sway of the nerves. As the flesh wastes in self-sacrifice, the penitent becomes 'all nerves', the mysteries of the female organization unveiled, or, to use another contemporary analogy, a piece of machinery whose faulty mechanism is exposed. The idea of a mechanism running down brings back to mind the clinical definition of neurasthenia and the physical laws which purported to explain the wear and tear upon the body caused by excessive mental and emotional demands.

Sue's acts of mortifying the flesh have important sexual connotations and are linked to her longing to free herself from her woman's body. It is too facile, though, as Penny Boumelha has rightly pointed out, to describe Sue Bridehead, with her self-confessed physical antipathies as 'sexless or frigid'.[81] Her quivering nervousness was consistent with the 'type of woman which had always had an attraction for me', wrote Hardy, namely, the intelligent, fastidious woman whose autonomy as to when and where she yielded herself only served to incite the passions of men, like Jude, who failed to discriminate between needful restraint and teasing refusal.[82] There is a self-consciousness in the novel about misconstruing Sue as 'cold-natured,—sexless' in her withholding of herself, a view she seeks to disabuse with subtle analysis. She is aware, in a way that her observers are not, of sexuality as a form of consciousness which is quite separate from the fixed, immutable categories in nature. What Jude simplistically sees as her 'curious unconsciousness of gender' (154) is precisely her more sophisticated consciousness of a distinction between the outward trappings which direct the common perception and an inward sense of a self-determined

---

[81] *Thomas Hardy and Women*, p. 142.
[82] *The Life of Thomas Hardy*, p. 272.

sexuality. Her point is made explicit in the same scene when, in the process of drying her clothes in Jude's lodgings after absconding from the college, she purports to forestall any misinterpretation that may be put on her hanging, disembodied garments with '[t]hey are only a woman's clothes—sexless cloth and linen' (150). Leaving aside the doubly portentous image presented by the hanging, lifeless garments—in respect of the dead children and of Sue's wasted flesh—Sue's distinction highlights the extent of the gap between their perceptions of sexual consciousness.

It is this capacity for making such distinctions which begins to fail as Sue's sickness dims her once shining intellect. Like Gwendolen Harleth, she loses the ability to distinguish between hierarchies of phenomena, and mistakenly believes that her own aberrant agency has precipitated events. Similarly, an air of unearthliness is observed in Sue, as it was in Gwendolen, from girlhood, and notably in a propensity for calling up the uncanny in their recitations by 'seeming to see things in the air' (114) which the more earthbound do not see. To Jude, Sue appears 'so ethereal a creature that her spirit could be seen trembling through her limbs' (195) and he measures his own blundering grossness against her unearthly quality:

It is more than this earthly wretch called Me deserves—you spirit, you disembodied creature, you dear, sweet, tantalizing phantom—hardly flesh at all; so that when I put my arms round you I almost expect them to pass through you as through air! (256–7)

Much is made of the contrast between this ethereal delicacy and Arabella's coarse fleshliness, but that is not to say that Sue's 'fastidiousness', as she herself calls it (221), is the polar opposite of Arabella's hearty availability. Jude is confused by the combination in Sue of the absence of 'animal passion' (272) and a refinement that is 'without inhuman sexlessness' (364). Paradoxically, it is that same enigmatic, elusive quality which defines her alienation. But instead of elevation into a realm of spiritual inaccessibility, her acts of disembodiment work only to bring about an estrangement more akin to the religious fanaticism traditionally associated with hysteria or even insanity.

The failure of individual intention is implicitly rooted in what Maudsley called the 'in-born structure'. Like Weismann's germ-plasm, this elusive material ensured the continuity not only of physiological heredity but of the 'weight of tradition, custom, habit, conformity' that presses 'like an atmosphere on every thought and feeling'.[83] When Sue, speaking on behalf of women, proclaims how '[w]e ought to be continually sacrificing ourselves on the altar of duty' (363), her atavistic recapitulation of that very conformity is confirmation that a once recalcitrant will has been forced to surrender to overmastering inherited moral mandates. Her acts of self-denial reach a macabre climax in the paroxysmal gesture of self-abasement in which she is reduced to 'a heap of black clothes . . . prostrate on the paving' before the Latin cross of St Silas's church (369). The vow to 'mortify the flesh', and 'to prick myself all over with pins and bleed out the badness that's in me!' (364) signifies on both religious and psychological levels. Renunciation and self-mutilation may be the prescribed acts of penance, but they also feature in contemporary medical ideas about a discrete female mind and the predominantly female disease of self-starvation, which was, in turn, linked to neurasthenia. Psychologically, Sue's punishing asceticism might be read as a retreat from the demands of mature reason and responsibility into the easy mechanics of ritual.

Although I have no grounds for claiming that Hardy's depiction of Sue's self-inflicted punishment was directly informed by medical knowledge, the description of his heroine's unrelenting excoriation of her womanly flesh to a pre-sexual, childlike condition consciously or unconsciously gestures towards the disease of anorexia. The term 'anorexia nervosa' is attributed to William Withey Gull, whose paper, 'Anorexia Nervosa (Apepsia Hysterica, Anorexia Hysterica)', given in 1873, makes reference to an earlier (1868) address by the author in which the disease was first named.[84] What is important about Gull's remarks in this context is the link he makes between the emaciation of the body and the 'mental perversity' of the young female sufferers.[85] In the absence of organic disease, their inanition, though

[83] *Natural Causes*, p. 208.

[84] William Withey Gull, 'Anorexia Nervosa (Apepsia Hysterica, Anorexia Hysterica)', in *Transactions of the Clinical Society of London*, 7 (London: Longmans, Green, 1874), pp. 22–8.

[85] Ibid., p. 25.

it may lead to death, is diagnosed as a function of an unsound mind requiring moral correction not medicine.[86] Clinical over-laps between anorexia, religious mania, and neurasthenia were widely corroborated in medical discourse, as were emerging psychological explanations of the malady which transformed the bodies of healthy young women into those of children. It is easy to see how this particular form of neurosis took on mean-ings of resistance to the Victorian norms of womanhood when the register of its symptoms is considered against the standard inventories of corporeal beauty and reproductive health which appeared in medical texts, many of which equalled Gissing's description of Mrs Morton in their effusive prose. The conjunc-tion of desirability and procreative potential was deeply ingrained in the nineteenth-century socio-medical sensibility. If the malady of excessive self-denial allowed its sufferers a measure of self-expression and control, to practitioners it signalled anything from perversity to mental derangement.

But the relationship of self-starvation to sexuality, and more particularly to the dynamics of power and control, was hinted at rather than stated. It is in denying her adult womanhood that Sue seems to have become 'a sort of fay, or sprite—not a woman!' (372).[87] There is a curious paradox in that her punish-ing regime reinforces volitional control even as it reduces her to a responding automaton. And another in an ethereality which is at once a defiance of a cultural ideal of nurturing womanhood and an extreme interpretation of the role of the domestic angel. 'I've wrestled and struggled, and fasted, and prayed. I have nearly brought my body into complete subjection' (410) Sue announces with perverse pride as she taunts Jude upon her return to Phillotson. On the morning of her remarriage, the change in her appearance is startlingly obvious to everyone:

---

[86] Gull's recommendations that anorexic patients should not be left to their own devices but coerced into complete rest and a nourishing diet sanction the view that the perverse female will must be broken in an enforced regimen. The main aim of the 'rest cure' was to fatten neurasthenic patients whose symptoms often included self-starvation.

[87] Helena Michie has argued that fasting is a means of purification which works by 'obliterating signs of sexuality' from the maturing female body. See *The Flesh Made Word: Female Figures and Women's Bodies* (Oxford: Oxford University Press, 1987), p. 21.

She had never in her life looked so much like the lily her name connoted as she did in that pallid morning light. Chastened, world-weary, remorseful, the strain on her nerves had preyed upon her flesh and bones, and she appeared smaller in outline than she had formerly done, though Sue had not been a large woman in her days of rudest health.   (389)

As the process of sacrificing herself 'on the altar of what she was pleased to call her principles' takes its toll, Sue's nerves are blatantly visible through a physical frame now so insubstantial that she has 'no body to speak of!' and seems, to Mrs Edlin, more like a 'sperrit' than a woman (415). But Sue does not achieve incorporeality despite her self-scourging. Instead, the stripping of the flesh exposes 'a mere cluster of nerves' from which 'all initiatory power' (379) has atrophied in the unremit-ting exhaustion of meeting the obligations to which she is phys-ically, psychologically, and intellectually averse.

   It is Jude's stubborn persistence in the principle of essential mental difference which exposes the inconsistencies in explana-tions of women's nervous disease. When he` acknowledges Sue as his 'guardian-angel' who alone keeps him from reverting to the condition of the 'pig that was washed turning back to his wallowing in the mire!' (373), we are reminded of George Romanes's assertion that a woman's mental structure is 'more refined: . . . further removed from the struggling instincts of the lower animals'.[88] Remarkably, then, Hardy's representation of Sue's nervous collapse exploits the very contradiction that Romanes stepped so cautiously around. Reduced to the primi-tive reflexes of a simple life form and, at the same time, refined to the point of unviability, Sue's nervous pathology spans the evolutionary scale.

Although neither Gissing nor Hardy uses the term 'neurasthe-nia', characteristic features of the disease are accurately drawn in their narratives. Alma and Sue are alike exhausted by the struggle to be different, to be 'new', to resist becoming enslaved by rules about sexual desire, marriage, and motherhood which have come to define the boundaries of normality. But Hardy's

---

[88] Hardy's allusion is also, of course, a biblical paraphrase: 'the sow is washed only to wallow in the mire' (2 Pet. 2: 22).

Sue is less easily accommodated into the formulaic pathologies of inherited morbidity, inferior mental capacity, or reckless disregard of the precious energy resources which women allegedly needed to conserve. Alma's nervous fatigue and death are attributed categorically to a rebellious and reckless nature which is unsympathetically allied to woman's supposed inaptitude for self-regulation. Sue's exhausted submission to the overmastering control of her nerves is, more equivocally, indicative both of personal failing and of a general dismay at the powerlessness of ideas in the stranglehold of biology. Her 'colossal inconsistency' is as much a function of the contradictions which confounded understanding of the interaction of heredity, environment, and nervous temperament as it is a reflection of her own inadequacy for the tasks she has set herself.

In the end, both women act to release the mind from the pain of present consciousness: Alma by resorting to her opium addiction, and Sue by surrender to a mind-numbing orthodoxy. Of Gissing's more explicitly accusatory narrative it might be argued that Alma's final act of recklessness (or rebellion) serves as confirmation of the moral weakness of which her sex was long suspected. No such simplistic satisfactions attach to Sue's capitulation, which, despite its hints of psychological instability linked to religious mania, is instigated more by her rigorous, if retrogressive, moral conscience than by mental impoverishment. And yet, physiologically speaking, it is the finer operations of her nerves, those which process the objective world into intellectual and moral consciousness, which are assumed by her to have become diseased. Her reversion to a state of nonvolitional, reactive functioning works at a number of interpretative levels. To Sue's own mind, retreat into passive submission is its own punishment for the folly of attempting to exceed or circumvent one's biological remit. Abandoning the struggle for social and intellectual emancipation, she assimilates the rhetoric of gender inequality of innate resources and settles back into the compliant conformity of the 'average' woman who 'never instigates, only responds' (372). When she burns her embroidered nightgown and takes the calico shift, she adopts the Christian way of healing the mind of its 'diseased' recalcitrance. But, importantly for Hardy, this strategy itself marks a backward turning, a reversion to the slavish forms of a primitive past. If, as Hardy had hypothesized, mental evolution had outgrown its 'corporeal conditions', nervous degeneration was symptomatic of the widening gap in which the mediating action of the nervous system had become impossibly overstretched and the fictional Sue, just like the hypothetical over-refined organism, reverts to a state of mental and bodily reflex function. Unlike Alma Rolfe, Sue lives on: stripped of intellect and of volitional power, a 'phantasmal, bodiless creature' (272) and ghostly cipher for the nervous degeneration which characterized the age.

Conclusion

Before the end of the century, psychiatric medicine was looking to define depression and nervous breakdown in terms far removed from the mechanistic analogies of wear and tear and drained resources. In part, the changes in interpretative and therapeutic methodology had to do with broader professional developments that were taking place; one of the most significant being the easing apart of psychology and neurology as medical specialisms.[1] The idea that neuroses might not, after all, arise from a disordered nervous system suggested a commitment to a concept of the mind as a distinct category for pathological investigation. Although psychoanalysis did not disregard social and environmental influences on patients' psychological states, it treated the processes of the mind independently, a procedure which the neurophysiologists of much of the century would have deprecated. As theories of neurosis rooted in the individual consciousness began to replace Victorian models of functional disorder, the disease of neurasthenia lost its cultural utility as a means of registering the failure of progressive individuals to meet the challenges they set for themselves, or of the nervously susceptible to withstand the rigours of modern life.[2] It was revived in the First World War narratives of shell shock such as Rebecca West's *The Return of the Soldier* (1918) but, by then, the social meanings of the disease had changed again.[3]

When psychoanalysts began to rewrite the textbook aetiologies of neuroses, their theories and their modes of treatment

[1] See Janet Oppenheim, *'Shattered Nerves': Doctors, Patients, and Depression in Victorian England* (New York: Oxford University Press, 1991) for a more extended discussion of these changes.

[2] For a critical evaluation of the uses of the term 'neurasthenia' in changing psychiatric and cultural climates, see 'The Concept of Neurasthenia', *International Journal of Psychiatry*, 9 (1970–1), 36–49.

[3] See Elaine Showalter, *The Female Madness: Women, Madness and English Culture, 1830–1980* (London: Virago, 1987. First published 1985) for a more extensive discussion of the re-appropriation of neurasthenia in the therapeutics of shell shock.

found many critics among the medical profession. Traditionalists remained profoundly suspicious. In 1910 Clifford Allbutt made it known how much he deplored the way in which modern psychiatric therapy completely ignored the medical criteria in neurasthenia and other nervous disorders when he lambasted its practitioners for turning the whole process of healing into a performative charade.[4] He strenuously denounced the unprofessional way in which some so-called 'analysts' were colluding with their patients in unreliable fictions of neurosis:

To me, possibly from personal prejudice, the recent introspective and confessional methods are odious. . . . We are hearing enough and to spare of suggestion—but what about the doctor's suggestion to his marionettes, these morbid women and effeminate men, enticed to heat up sophisticated autobiographies, egotisms, and fictions? . . . For these secret introspective dramas, inflamed by reminiscent curiosity, are more than half factitious; and thirst for experience is confused with frailty of morals. . . . The emphasis laid by many authors on the sexual passion beyond, and even to the neglect of other emotions, and their curious pursuit into remotest recesses of its inventions and lusts, seem to me in method false, and to engender sophistry and pruriency.[5]

Allbutt's critique is instructive in its indication of how far concepts of neurosis had moved from a medicine of symptoms in which doctors diagnosed aberrant behaviour according to fixed categories of disease. In its place, the nature of the disorder, its cause, manifestation, and prognosis, came to be seen as individual, peculiar to the sufferer, different in every case. Effectively, the new psychology collapsed many of the boundaries between health and disease, and between patient and practitioner, by turning the process of diagnosis and treatment into a shifting sand of perception and interpretation. In the process of analysis, neuroses acquired meanings only in the transition from their allegedly forgotten or repressed origins into consciousness.

---

[4] Sigmund Freud himself, of course, began his career in medicine as a neurologist and for many years was committed to the belief that neuroses stemmed from physiological dysfunction of hereditary origin.

[5] Clifford Allbutt, 'Neurasthenia', in T. C. Allbutt and Humphry Davy Rolleston (eds.), *A System of Medicine*, 2nd edn., 9 vols. (London: Macmillan, 1905–11), viii, pp. 759–60.

Consciousness itself had taken on new dimensions although, as critics have pointed out, we would be wrong in thinking that Sigmund Freud was the first to conceive of the 'unconscious' as the submerged, but continuously operative, aspect of the conscious. The ideas discussed in the first part of Chapter 3 of this book are clear evidence that the workings of the unconscious mind and the interpretation of dreams and delusions were the subjects of serious scientific investigation many decades before Freud. In other respects, too, Freud's analyses of psychopathological states drew heavily upon earlier medical knowledge and practice. There are undoubted similarities between Freud's symbolism and the 'association of ideas' models of how the mind works which had been developed around the turn of the nineteenth century, although, in fact, they can be traced back to classical times. Allbutt's dismay about the over-emphasis on the sexual passion and the 'curious pursuit into remotest recesses of its inventions and lusts' calls back to mind earlier controversies about the disputed existence of female sexual passion, the social necessity to repress that which reputedly did not exist, and the conflicting warnings as to the morbid consequences of both repression and expression. Not new either are what we may think of as relatively recent questions about its therapeutic efficacy, as Allbutt's invective clearly shows. If psychoanalysis brought a new fluency to the interpretation and expression of pathological states, it was scientifically unoriginal. Indeed many years earlier G. H. Lewes had observed of all the so-called 'new' mental sciences that they seized upon the cultural sensibilities of the day to frame their theories and methodologies accordingly.[6] As a literary critic turned amateur neurophysiologist, Lewes was in a better position than many to comment on the relationship between observable phenomena and the ways in which those phenomena are interpreted and represented. For the positivist physicians of the second half of the nineteenth century, the hope was that the passions, like all of mental life, would one day be understood in terms of measurable changes in cerebral neurones rather than being attributed somewhat arbitrarily to designated areas of the brain. Few, however, went so far as to claim with confidence

[6] *The Foundations of a Creed*, vol. 1 (London: Trübner, 1874).

that 'mind' was a meaningless concept if separated from the activity of the brain. In our own time, the search for a physiological elucidation of the nature of mental life continues as neurologists of the twenty-first century probe the organ of the brain for the mysteries of consciousness itself.

Select Bibliography

NOVELS AND OTHER PRIMARY LITERARY SOURCES

Allen, Grant, *The Woman Who Did* (London: John Lane, 1895).

Arnold, Matthew, 'The Scholar-Gipsy' (1853), in Kenneth Allott (ed.), *The Poems of Matthew Arnold* (London: Longmans, 1965).

Brontë, Anne, *Agnes Grey* (1847), ed. by Angeline Goreau (Harmondsworth: Penguin, 1988).

Brontë, Charlotte, *Shirley* (1849), ed. by Herbert Rosengarten and Margaret Smith (Oxford: Oxford University Press, 1979; with intro. by Margaret Smith, 1981).

——, *Villette* (1853), ed. by Margaret Smith and Herbert Rosengarten (Oxford: Oxford University Press, 1984; with intro. by Margaret Smith, 1990).

——, *The Professor* (1857), ed. by Heather Glen (Harmondsworth: Penguin, 1989).

Collins, Wilkie, *Basil* (1852), ed. by Dorothy Goldman (Oxford: Oxford University Press, 1990).

——, 'Mad Monkton'(1852), repr. in *Mad Monkton and Other Stories*, ed. by Norman Page (Oxford: Oxford University Press, 1994).

——, *The Woman in White* (1860), ed. by John Sutherland (Oxford: Oxford University Press, 1996).

——, *Heart and Science: A Story of the Present Time* (1883), ed. by Steve Farmer (Peterborough, Ontario: Broadview Press, 1996).

Dickens, Charles, *Bleak House* (1853), ed. by Norman Page, with intro. by J. Hillis Miller (Harmondsworth: Penguin, 1971).

——, *Little Dorrit* (1855–7), ed. by Stephen Wall and Helen Small (Harmondsworth: Penguin, 1998).

——, *Great Expectations* (1860–1), ed. by Edgar Rosenberg (New York: W. W. Norton, 1999).

——, *Our Mutual Friend* (1864–5), ed. by Stephen Gill (Harmondsworth: Penguin, 1971).

Eliot, George, 'The Lifted Veil' (1859), ed. by Helen Small (Oxford: Oxford University Press, 1999).

——, *The Lifted Veil*, with a new Afterword by Beryl Gray (London: Virago, 1985).

Eliot, George, *Daniel Deronda* (1876), ed. by Terence Cave (Harmondsworth: Penguin, 1995).

——, *The George Eliot Letters*, ed. by Gordon S. Haight, 9 vols. (London: Oxford University Press, 1954–78).

Gaskell, Elizabeth, *Cousin Phillis* (1864), ed. by Peter Keating (Harmondsworth: Penguin, 1976).

Gilman, Charlotte Perkins, 'The Yellow Wallpaper', first published in *New England Magazine* (1892), repr. in Ann J. Lane, *The Charlotte Perkins Gilman Reader* (New York: Pantheon, 1980).

Gissing, George, *The Whirlpool* (1897), ed. by Patrick Parrinder (London: Harvester, 1977).

Grand, Sarah, *The Heavenly Twins* (1893), ed. by Carol A. Senf (Michigan: University of Michigan Press, 1992).

Hardy, Thomas, *The Return of the Native* (1878), ed. by George Woodcock (Harmondsworth: Penguin, 1978).

——, *Jude the Obscure* (1895), ed. by Patricia Ingham (Oxford: Oxford University Press, 1985).

——, *The Literary Notebooks of Thomas Hardy*, ed. by Lennart Björk, 2 vols. (London: Macmillan, 1985).

Le Fanu, Sheridan, *In a Glass Darkly* (1872), ed. by Robert Tracy (New York: Oxford: Oxford University Press, 1993).

MacDonald, George, *Adela Cathcart* (1864) (Whitethorn, Calif.: Johannesen, 1994).

Martineau, Harriet, *Deerbrook* (1839), with intro. by Gaby Weiner (New York: The Dial Press, 1983).

Meredith, George, *The Ordeal of Richard Feverel*, new edn. (London: Chapman and Hall, 1894).

Patmore, Coventry, 'The Angel in the House' (London: George Bell, 1887).

Poe, Edgar Allan, *Poetry and Tales*, ed. by Patrick F. Quinn (New York: Literary Classics of the United States, 1984).

Ruskin, John, *Sesame and Lilies* (1865), 14th edn. (London: George Allen, 1894).

Symons, Arthur, 'Nerves', in *London Nights* (1895), repr. in *The Faber Book of Twentieth Century Verse*, new edn., rev. by John Heath-Stubbs and David Wright (London: Faber, 1953).

Wood, Mrs Henry, *East Lynne* (1861), ed. by Stevie Davies (London: Dent, 1984).

PRIMARY MEDICAL SOURCES, SOCIAL COMMENTARY, AND
OTHER NON-FICTIONAL MATERIAL

Acton, William, *The Functions and Disorders of the Reproductive Organs in Childhood, in Youth, in Adult Age and in Advanced Life,*

Considered in Their Physiological, Social and Moral Relations, 4th edn. (London: John Churchill, 1865).

Allbutt, T. Clifford, *On Visceral Neuroses* (London: John Churchill, 1884).

——, 'Nervous Diseases and Modern Life', *Contemporary Review*, 67 (1895), 210–31.

——, 'Neurasthenia', in T. C. Allbutt and Humphry Davy Rolleston (eds.), *A System of Medicine*, 2nd edn., 9 vols. (London: Macmillan, 1905–11), viii. pp. 727–89.

Anderson, Elizabeth Garrett, 'Sex in Mind and Education: A Reply', *Fortnightly Review*, n.s. 15 (May, 1874), 582–94.

Anon., 'Woman in Her Psychological Relations', *Journal of Psychological Medicine and Mental Pathology*, 4 (1851), 18–50.

Bain, Alexander, *Mind and Body; the Theories of Their Relation* (London: Henry S. King, 1873).

Barlow, John, *On Man's Power Over Himself to Prevent or Control Insanity* (London: William Pickering, 1843).

Bernard, Claude, *Lectures in Animal Heat* (Paris: J-B. Ballière, 1876).

——, *Lectures in Diabetes and Animal Glycogenesis* (Paris: J-B. Ballière, 1877).

Brewster, David, 'Mental Physiology', *North British Review*, 22 (1854), 179–224.

Burrows, George Man, *On Disorders of the Cerebral Circulation and on the Connection Between Affections of the Brain and Diseases of the Heart* (London: Longman, Brown, Green, and Longmans, 1846).

Carpenter, William Benjamin, *Principles of Human Physiology*, 4th edn. (London: John Churchill, 1853).

Carter, Robert Brudenell, *On the Pathology and Treatment of Hysteria* (London: John Churchill, 1853).

Cheyne, George, *The English Malady or a Treatise of Nervous Diseases of All Kinds as Spleen, Vapours, Lowness of Spirits, Hypochondriacal and Hysterical Distempers* (London: Strahan and Leake, 1733).

Clouston, T. S., *Clinical Lectures on Mental Diseases*, 2nd edn. (London: John Churchill, 1887).

Cobbe, Frances Power, 'Unconscious Cerebration: A Psychological Study', *Macmillan's Magazine*, 23 (1870), 24–37.

Comte, Auguste, *The Positive Philosophy*, trans. by Harriet Martineau, 2 vols. (London: Trübner, 1875).

Copland, James, *A Dictionary of Practical Medicine: comprising general pathology, the nature and treatment of diseases, morbid structures, and the disorders especially incidental to the climates, to the sex, and to the different epochs of life &c.*, 3 vols.

(London: Longman, Brown, Green, Longmans, & Roberts, 1858).

Crichton-Browne, James, 'Education and the Nervous System', in Malcolm Morris (ed.), *The Book of Health* (London: Cassell, 1884), pp. 269–380.

Darwin, Charles, *The Origin of Species by Means of Natural Selection; or, The Preservation of Favoured Races in the Struggle for Life* (1859), ed. by J. W. Burrow (Harmondsworth: Penguin, 1968)

——, *The Descent of Man, and Selection in Relation to Sex* (1871), 2nd edn. (London: John Murray, 1883).

Day, George Edward, 'Louise Lateau: A Biological Study', Art.14, *Neurology*, [n.d.], 488–98.

Donkin, H. B., 'Hysteria', in D. H. Tuke (ed.), *A Dictionary of Psychological Medicine*, 2 vols. (London: John Churchill, 1892), i, pp. 618–27.

Dowse, Thomas Stretch, *On Brain and Nerve Exhaustion (Neurasthenia), and on the Nervous Sequelæ of Influenza* (London: Baillière, Tindall, and Cox, 1894).

Duffey, Eliza B., *What Women Should Know: A Woman's Book About Women. Containing Practical Information for Wives and Mothers* (Philadelphia: [n.pub.], 1873).

Duncan, George, *The Various Theories of the Relation of Mind and Brain* (London: Trübner, 1869).

Elliotson, John, *Human Physiology*, 5th edn. (London: Longmans, 1840).

Ellis, Sarah Stickney, *The Women of England: Their Social Duties and Domestic Habits* (London: Fisher, 1838).

Forbes, J., Tweedie, A., and Conolly, J. (eds.), *The Cyclopaedia of Practical Medicine*, 4 vols. (London: Sherwood, Gilbert, Piper *et al.*, 1833–5).

Gull, William Withey, 'Anorexia Nervosa (Apepsia Hysterica, Anorexia Hysterica)', in *Transactions of the Clinical Society of London*, 7 (London: Longmans, Green, 1874), pp. 22–8.

Hardy, Thomas, Art.viii, 'The Tree of Knowledge', *New Review*, 10 (1894), 675–90 (p. 681).

Holland, Henry, *Medical Notes and Reflections*, 3rd edn. (London: Longman, Brown, Green, and Longmans, 1855).

——, *Chapters on Mental Physiology*, 2nd edn. (London: Longman, Brown, Green, Longmans, & Roberts, 1858).

Laycock, Thomas, *A Treatise on the Nervous Diseases of Women* (London: Longman, Orme, Brown, Green, and Longmans, 1840).

Lewes, G. H., 'The Lady Novelists', *Westminster Review*, o.s.58 (1852), 129–41.

——, *The Physiology of Common Life*, 2 vols. (Edinburgh: Blackwood, 1859–60).

——, *Problems of Life and Mind*, 3 series: *The Foundations of a Creed*, 2 vols. (1874, 1875); *The Physical Basis of Mind* (1877). *The Study of Psychology* (1879), and *Problems of Life and Mind*, ser. 3, vol. 2, rev. by Michael Foster and James Sully, were published posthumously (London: Trübner, 1879).

Lewis, William Bevan, *A Textbook of Mental Diseases* (London: Charles Griffin, 1889).

Maudsley, Henry, 'Memoir of the Late John Conolly, M.D.', *Journal of Mental Science*, 12 (1866), 151–74.

——, *Body and Mind: An Enquiry Into Their Connection and Mutual Influence, Specially in Reference to Mental Disorders*, being the Gulstonian Lectures for 1870 (London: Macmillan, 1870).

——, 'Sex in Mind and in Education', *Fortnightly Review*, n.s. 15 (April, 1874), 466–83.

——, *The Physiology of Mind*, rev. edn. of *The Physiology and Pathology of Mind* (London: Macmillan, 1876).

——, *Natural Causes and Supernatural Seemings* (London: Kegan Paul, Trench, 1886).

Michelet, Jules, *La Femme* (1859), Préface de Thérèse Moreau (Paris: Flammarion, 1981).

Millingen, J. G., *Mind and Matter, Illustrated by Considerations on Heredity, Insanity, and the Influence of Temperament in the Development of the Passions* (London: H. Hurst, 1847).

Nordau, Max, *Degeneration* (1892), trans. from 2nd edn. (London: Heinemann, 1913).

[Oliphant, Margaret], 'Sensation Novels', *Blackwood's Magazine*, 102 (1867), 257–80.

Paget, James, 'Sexual Hypochondriasis' (1870), in Howard Marsh (ed.), *Clinical Lectures and Essays*, 2nd edn. (London: Longmans, Green, 1879), pp. 275–98.

Prichard, J. C., *On the Different Forms of Insanity in Relation to Jurisprudence* (London: Hippolyte Ballière, 1842).

Reid, John, *Essays on Hypochondriasis*, 2nd edn. (London: Longman, Hurst, Rees, Orme, and Brown, 1821).

Romanes, George J., 'Mental Differences Between Men and Women', *Nineteenth Century*, 21 (1887), 654–72.

Skey, F. C., *Lectures on Hysteria* (London: Longmans, Green, Reader, & Dyer, 1867).

Spencer, Herbert, *The Principles of Psychology*, 2 vols. (London: Williams and Norgate, 1855).

——, *The Principles of Sociology* (1876), 3rd edn., 3 vols. (London: Williams and Norgate, 1904).

Sully, James, *Sensation and Intuition: Studies in Psychology and Aesthetics* (London: Henry S. King, 1874).

Tooley, Sarah A., 'The Woman Question: An Interview with Madame Sarah Grand', *The Humanitarian*, ed. by Victoria Woodhull Martin, 8/3 (March, 1896), 160–9.

Trotter, Thomas, *Medicina Nautica: An Essay on the Diseases of Seamen*, 3 vols. (London: Longman, Hurst, Rees, and Orme, 1804; vol. i being a 2nd edn. of the 1797 single volume).

——, *A View of the Nervous Temperament, Being a Practical Enquiry into the Increasing Prevalence, Prevention, and Treatment of Those Diseases Commonly Called Nervous* (London: Longman, Hurst, Rees, Orme, and Brown, 1807).

Tuke, D. H. (ed.), *A Dictionary of Psychological Medicine*, 2 vols. (London: John Churchill, 1892).

Weismann, August, *Essays Upon Heredity and Kindred Biological Problems*, 2 vols. (Oxford: Clarendon Press, 1889–92).

SECONDARY SOURCES

Ashton, Rosemary, *G. H. Lewes: A Life* (Oxford: Clarendon Press, 1991).

Bailey, Margery (ed.), *Boswell's Column: Being his Seventy Contributions to THE LONDON MAGAZINE under the Pseudonym THE HYPOCHONDRIACK from 1777 to 1783 here First Printed in Book Form in England* (London: William Kimber, 1951).

Bailin, Miriam, *The Sickroom in Victorian Fiction: The Art of Being Ill* (Cambridge: Cambridge University Press, 1994).

Baker, William, *The George Eliot–George Henry Lewes Library: An Annotated Catalogue of Their Books at Dr. Williams's Library, London* (New York: Garland Publishing, 1977).

Beer, Gillian, *Darwin's Plots: Evolutionary Narrative in Darwin, George Eliot and Nineteenth-Century Fiction* (London: Ark Paperbacks, 1985. First published 1983).

——, 'Origins and Oblivion in Victorian Narrative', in Ruth Bernard Yeazell (ed.), *Sex, Politics and Science in the Nineteenth-Century Novel*, Selected Papers From the English Institute, 1983–4 (Baltimore: Johns Hopkins University Press, 1986), pp. 63–87.

Beer, Patricia, *Reader, I Married Him* (London: Macmillan, 1974).

Benton, Graham, ' "And Dying Thus Around Us Every Day": Pathology, Ontology and the Discourse of the Diseased Body, A Study of Illness and Contagion in *Bleak House*', *Dickens Quarterly*, 11 (1994), 69–80.

Boumelha, Penny, *Thomas Hardy and Women: Sexual Ideology and Narrative Form* (Brighton: Harvester Press, 1982).

Bynum, W. F., 'The Nervous Patient in Eighteenth and Nineteenth-Century Britain: the Psychiatric Origins of British Neurology', in W. F. Bynum, Roy Porter, and Michael Shepherd (eds.), *The Anatomy of Madness: Essays in the History of Psychiatry*, 3 vols. (London: Tavistock Publications, 1985), i, pp. 89–102.

Canguilhem, Georges, *The Normal and the Pathological*, intro. by Michel Foucault, trans. by Carolyn R. Fawcett (New York: Zone Books, 1989).

Carroll, David, *George Eliot and the Conflict of Interpretations: A Reading of the Novels* (Cambridge: Cambridge University Press, 1992).

Chase, Karen, *Eros and Psyche: The Representation of Personality in Charlotte Brontë, Charles Dickens, and George Eliot* (London: Methuen, 1984).

Chatel, John, and Peele, Roger, 'The Concept of Neurasthenia', *International Journal of Psychiatry*, 9 (1970–1), 36–49.

Cixous, Hélène and Clément, Catherine, *The Newly Born Woman*, trans. by Betsy Wing (Manchester: Manchester University Press, 1986. First published as *La Jeune Née*, Paris, 1975).

Clark, Michael, ' "Morbid Introspection": Unsoundness of Mind, and British Psychological Medicine, *c*.1830–*c*.1900', in W. F. Bynum, Roy Porter, and Michael Shepherd (eds.), *The Anatomy of Madness: Essays in the History of Psychiatry*, 3 vols. (London: Tavistock Publications, 1985), iii, pp. 71–101.

Cohen, Ed, *Talk on the Wilde Side: Toward a Genealogy of a Discourse on Male Sexualities* (London: Routledge, 1993).

Cooter, Roger, *The Cultural Meaning of Popular Science: Phrenology and the Organization of Consent in Nineteenth-Century Britain* (Cambridge: Cambridge University Press, 1984).

Cosslett, Tess, *Woman to Woman: Female Friendship in Victorian Fiction* (Brighton: Harvester Press, 1988).

Coustillas, Pierre (ed.), *London and the Life of Literature in Late Victorian England: The Diary of George Gissing, Novelist* (Brighton: Harvester Press, 1978).

Cox, R. G. (ed.), *Thomas Hardy: The Critical Heritage* (London: Routledge & Kegan Paul, 1970).

Cunningham, Gail, *The New Woman and the Victorian Novel* (London: Macmillan, 1978).

Dale, Peter A., 'Thomas Hardy and the Best Consummation Possible', in John Christie and Sally Shuttleworth (eds.), *Nature Transfigured: Science and Literature, 1700–1900* (Manchester: Manchester University Press, 1989), pp. 201–21.

Daly, K., 'A Study of Nostalgia and Cosmopolitanism in Relation to the Works of Byron', unpub. Ph.D. thesis (University of Leeds, 1996).

Delamont, Sara, and Duffin, Lorna (eds.), *The Nineteenth-Century Woman: Her Cultural and Physical World* (London: Croom Helm, 1978).

Dijkstra, Bram, *Idols of Perversity: Fantasies of Feminine Evil in Fin-de-Siècle Culture* (New York: Oxford University Press, 1986).

Drinka, George Frederick, *The Birth of Neurosis: Myth, Malady, and the Victorians* (New York: Simon and Schuster, 1984).

During, Simon, 'The Strange Case of Monomania: Patriarchy in Literature, Murder in *Middlemarch*, Drowning in *Daniel Deronda*', *Representations*, 23 (1988), 86–104.

Eagleton, Terry, *Myths of Power: A Marxist Study of the Brontës* (London: Macmillan, 1975).

——, 'Power and Knowledge in "The Lifted Veil" ', *Literature and History*, 9 (1983), 52–61.

Ehrenreich, Barbara, and English, Deirdre, *Complaints and Disorders: The Sexual Politics of Sickness* (London: Writers and Readers Publishing Co-operative, 1976. First published 1973).

Flint, Kate, 'Blood, Bodies, and *The Lifted Veil*', *Nineteenth-Century Literature*, 51/4 (1997), 455–73.

Foucault, Michel, *The Birth of the Clinic: An Archaeology of Medical Perception*, trans. by A. M. Sheridan (London: Tavistock Publications, 1973. First published 1963).

——, *The History of Sexuality*, vol. i, trans. by Robert Hurley (Harmondsworth: Penguin, 1981. First published 1976).

Gallivan, Patricia, 'Science and Art in *Jude the Obscure*', in Anne Smith (ed.), *The Novels of Thomas Hardy* (London: Vision Press, 1979), pp. 126–44.

Gay, Peter, *The Bourgeois Experience: Victoria to Freud*, 2 vols. (New York: Oxford University Press, 1986).

Gilman, Sander L., *Seeing the Insane: A Cultural History of Madness and Art in the Western World* (New York: Wiley, 1982).

Goldstein, Jan, *Console and Classify: The French Psychiatric Profession in the Nineteenth Century* (Cambridge: Cambridge University Press, 1987).

——, 'The Uses of Male Hysteria: Medical and Literary Discourse in Nineteenth-Century France', *Representations*, 34 (1991), 134–65.

Gray, B. M., 'Pseudoscience and George Eliot's "The Lifted Veil" ', *Nineteenth-Century Fiction*, 36 (1982), 407–23.

Greenslade, William, *Degeneration, Culture and the Novel 1880–1940* (Cambridge: Cambridge University Press, 1994).

Grylls, David, *The Paradox of Gissing* (London: Allen & Unwin, 1986).

Haight, Gordon S., *George Eliot: A Biography* (Oxford: Oxford University Press, 1968).

Haller, John S., and Haller, Robin M., *The Physician and Sexuality in Victorian America* (Chicago: University of Illinois Press, 1974).

Hardy, Barbara, Introduction to George Eliot, *Daniel Deronda* (Harmondsworth: Penguin, 1967).

Hardy, F. E., *The Life of Thomas Hardy 1840–1928* (London: Macmillan, 1962).

Jacobus, Mary, Keller, Evelyn Fox, and Shuttleworth, Sally (eds.), *Body/Politics: Women and the Discourses of Science* (London: Routledge, 1990).

Jordanova, Ludmilla, *Sexual Visions: Images of Gender in Science and Medicine Between the Eighteenth and Twentieth Centuries* (Hemel Hempstead: Harvester Wheatsheaf, 1989).

Kaplan, Fred, *Dickens and Mesmerism: The Hidden Springs of Fiction* (Princeton, NJ: Princeton University Press, 1975).

Langland, Elizabeth, 'Nobody's Angels: Domestic Ideology and Middle-Class Women in the Victorian Novel', *PMLA*, 107 (1992), 290–304.

Ledger, Sally, *The New Woman: Fiction and Feminism at the Fin de Siècle* (Manchester: Manchester University Press, 1997).

Maynard, John, *Charlotte Brontë and Sexuality* (Cambridge: Cambridge University Press, 1984).

Menke, Richard, 'Fiction as Vivisection: G. H. Lewes and George Eliot', *ELH*, 67/2 (2000), 617–53.

Michie, Helena, *The Flesh Made Word: Female Figures and Women's Bodies* (Oxford: Oxford University Press, 1987).

Moglen, Helene, *Charlotte Brontë: The Self Conceived* (New York: W. W. Norton, 1976).

Mort, Frank, *Dangerous Sexualities: Medico-Moral Politics in England Since 1830* (London: Routledge and Kegan Paul, 1987).

Morton, Peter, *The Vital Science: Biology and the Literary Imagination, 1860–1900* (London: Allen & Unwin, 1984).

Nead, Lynda, *Myths of Sexuality: Representations of Women in Victorian Britain* (Oxford: Blackwell, 1988).

Nestor, Pauline, *Charlotte Brontë* (London: Macmillan, 1983).

Oppenheim, Janet, *'Shattered Nerves': Doctors, Patients, and Depression in Victorian England* (New York: Oxford University Press, 1991).

Paxton, Nancy, *George Eliot and Herbert Spencer: Feminism, Evolutionism, and the Reconstruction of Gender* (Princeton, NJ: Princeton University Press, 1991).

Pearce, Lynne, *Woman, Image, Text: Readings in Pre-Raphaelite Art and Literature* (Hemel Hempstead: Harvester Wheatsheaf, 1991).

Peterson, Audrey C., 'Brain Fever in Nineteenth-Century Literature: Fact and Fiction', *Victorian Studies*, 19 (1976), 445–64.

Peterson, M. Jeanne, *The Medical Profession in Mid-Victorian London* (Berkeley, Calif.: University of California Press, 1978).
——, 'Dr. Acton's Enemy: Medicine, Sex, and Society in Victorian England', *Victorian Studies*, 29 (1986), 569–90.
Pick, Daniel, *Faces of Degeneration: A European Disorder, c.1848–c.1918* (Cambridge: Cambridge University Press, 1989).
Poovey, Mary, 'Speaking of the Body: Mid-Victorian Constructions of Female Desire', in Mary Jacobus, Evelyn Fox Keller, and Sally Shuttleworth (eds.), *Body/Politics: Women and the Discourses of Science* (New York: Routledge, 1990), pp. 29–46.
Porter, Roy, *Disease, Medicine and Society in England 1550–1860* (London: Macmillan, 1987).
——, *Mind-Forg'd Manacles: A History of Madness in England from the Restoration to the Regency* (Cambridge, Mass.: Harvard University Press, 1987).
Pykett, Lyn, *The 'Improper Feminine': The Women's Sensation Novel and the New Woman Writing* (London: Routledge, 1992).
Rosenberg, Charles E., 'Body and Mind in Nineteenth-Century Medicine: Some Clinical Origins of the Neurosis Construct', *Bulletin of the History of Medicine*, 63 (1989), 185–97.
Rothfield, Lawrence, *Vital Signs: Medical Realism in Nineteenth-Century Fiction* (Princeton, NJ: Princeton University Press, 1992).
Russett, Cynthia Eagle, *Sexual Science: The Victorian Construction of Womanhood* (Cambridge, Mass.: Harvard University Press, 1989).
Schiller, Francis, *A Möbius Strip: Fin-de-Siècle Neuropsychiatry and Paul Möbius* (Berkeley, Calif.: University of California Press, 1982).
Shorter, Edward, *From Paralysis to Fatigue: A History of Psychosomatic Illness in the Modern Era* (New York: Free Press, 1992).
Showalter, Elaine, *A Literature of Their Own: British Women Novelists from Brontë to Lessing* (Princeton, NJ.: Princeton University Press, 1977).
——, *The Female Malady: Women, Madness, and English Culture, 1830–1980* (London: Virago, 1987. First published 1985).
——, *Sexual Anarchy: Gender and Culture at the Fin de Siècle* (London: Virago, 1992).
Shuttleworth, Sally, *George Eliot and Nineteenth-Century Science: The Make-Believe of a Beginning* (Cambridge: Cambridge University Press, 1984).
——, 'Preaching to the Nerves: Psychological Disorder in Sensation Fiction', in M. Benjamin (ed.), *A Question of Identity: Women, Science and Literature* (New Brunswick, NJ: Rutgers University Press, 1993), pp. 192–244.
——, *Charlotte Brontë and Victorian Psychology* (Cambridge: Cambridge University Press, 1996).

Sloan, John, *George Gissing: The Cultural Challenge* (London: Macmillan, 1989).

Small, Helen, *Love's Madness: Medicine, the Novel, and Female Insanity 1800–1865* (Oxford: Clarendon Press, 1996).

Taylor, Jenny Bourne, *In the Secret Theatre of Home: Wilkie Collins, Sensation Narrative, and Nineteenth-Century Psychology* (London: Routledge, 1988).

——, 'Obscure Recesses: Locating the Victorian Unconscious', in J. B. Bullen (ed.), *Writing and Victorianism* (New York: Longman, 1997).

Tingle, C. M. 'Symptomatic Writings: Prefigurations of Freudian Theories and Models of the Mind in the Fiction of Sheridan Le Fanu, Wilkie Collins, and George Eliot', unpublished Ph.D. thesis (University of Leeds, 2000).

Todd, John, and Ashworth, Lawrence, *"The House": Wakefield Asylum 1818–. . .* (Wakefield: the authors, 1993).

Tosh, John, *A Man's Place: Masculinity and the Middle-Class Home in Victorian England* (New Haven and London: Yale University Press, 1999).

Turner, Trevor, 'Henry Maudsley: Psychiatrist, Philosopher, and Entrepreneur', in W. F. Bynum, Roy Porter, and Michael Shepherd (eds.), *The Anatomy of Madness: Essays in the History of Psychiatry*, 3 vols. (London: Tavistock Publications, 1985), iii, pp. 151–89.

Veith, Ilza, *Hysteria: The History of a Disease* (Chicago: University of Chicago Press, 1965).

Vickery, Amanda, 'Golden Age to Separate Spheres? A Review of the Categories and Chronology of English Women's History', *The Historical Journal*, 36, 2 (1993), 383–414.

Vrettos, Athena, *Somatic Fictions: Imagining Illness in Victorian Culture* (Stanford: Stanford University Press, 1995).

Williams, A. Susan, *The Rich Man and the Diseased Poor in Early Victorian Literature* (London: Macmillan, 1987).

Yeazell, Ruth Bernard, (ed.), *Sex, Politics, and Science in the Nineteenth-Century Novel*, Selected Papers from the English Institute, 1983–4 (Baltimore: Johns Hopkins University Press, 1986).

Young, Robert M., *Mind, Brain, and Adaptation in the Nineteenth Century: Cerebral Localization and its Biological Context from Gall to Ferrier* (Oxford: Clarendon Press, 1970).

Zimmerman, Bonnie, 'Gwendolen Harleth and "The Girl of the Period" ', in Anne Smith (ed.), *George Eliot: Centenary Essays and an Unpublished Fragment* (London: Vision Press, 1980), pp. 196–217.

Index